T0327432

Injectable Fillers

Injectable Fillers: Facial Shaping and Contouring

Second Edition

EDITED BY

Derek H. Jones, MD

Medical Director
Skin Care and Laser Physicians of Beverly Hills
Los Angeles, CA
USA

Arthur Swift, MD

Plastic Surgeon
The Westmount Institute of Plastic Surgery
Montreal, QC
Canada

WILEY Blackwell

Registered Office(s)
John Wiley & Sons, Inc., 111 River Street, Hoboken, NJ 07030, USA
John Wiley & Sons Ltd, The Atrium, Southern Gate, Chichester, West Sussex, PO19 8SQ, UK

Editorial Office
9600 Garsington Road, Oxford, OX4 2DQ, UK

For details of our global editorial offices, customer services, and more information about Wiley products visit us at www.wiley.com.

Wiley also publishes its books in a variety of electronic formats and by print-on-demand. Some content that appears in standard print versions of this book may not be available in other formats.

Library of Congress Cataloging-in-Publication Data

Names: Jones, Derek H., 1965– editor. | Swift, Arthur, editor.
Title: Injectable fillers : facial shaping and contouring / edited by Derek H. Jones, Arthur Swift.
Description: Second edition. | Hoboken, NJ : Wiley-Blackwell, 2019. | Includes bibliographical
    references and index. |
Identifiers: LCCN 2018048131 (print) | LCCN 2018049205 (ebook) | ISBN 9781119046967
    (Adobe PDF) | ISBN 9781119046950 (ePub) | ISBN 9781119046943 (hardcover)
Subjects: | MESH: Face–surgery | Cosmetic Techniques | Injections–methods
Classification: LCC RD119.5.F33 (ebook) | LCC RD119.5.F33 (print) | NLM WE 705 |
    DDC 617.5/2059–dc23
LC record available at https://lccn.loc.gov/2018048131

Cover Design: Wiley
Cover Image: ©RomoloTavani/iStockphoto

Set in 9.5/13pt Meridien by SPi Global, Pondicherry, India

10 9 8 7 6 5 4 3 2 1

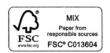

Contents

List of Contributors

Frederick C. Beddingfield, III MD, PhD
Sienna Biopharmaceuticals, Westlake Village, CA, USA

Katie Beleznay MD, FRCPC, FAAD
Carruthers & Humphrey Cosmetic Dermatology and University of British Columbia, Vancouver, British Columbia, Canada

Jeanette M. Black MD
Skin Care and Laser Physicians of Beverly Hills, Los Angeles, CA, USA

Sebastian Cotofana MD
Skin Care and Laser Physicians of Beverly Hills, Los Angeles, CA, USA
and
Department of Medical Education, Albany Medical College, Albany, NY, USA

Claudio DeLorenzi MD
The DeLorenzi Clinic, Kitchener, Ontario, Canada

Shannon Humphrey MD, FRCPC, FAAD
Carruthers & Humphrey Cosmetic Dermatology and University of British Columbia, Vancouver, British Columbia, Canada

Derek H. Jones MD
Skin Care and Laser Physicians of Beverly Hills, Los Angeles, CA, USA

Krishnan M. Kapoor MD
Fortis Hospital, Mohali, Punjab, India
and
Anticlock Clinic, Chandigarh, India

B. Kent Remington MD
Remington Laser Dermatology Centre, Calgary, Canada

Paul F. Lizzul MD, PhD, MPH, MBA
Sienna Biopharmaceuticals, Westlake Village, CA, USA

Ardalan Minokadeh MD, PhD
Skin Care and Laser Physicians of Beverly Hills, Los Angeles, CA, USA

Amir Moradi MD
Moradi M.D., Vista, CA, USA

Tatjana Pavicic MD
Private Practice for Dermatology and Aesthetics, Munich, Germany

Herve Raspaldo MD
Private Practice Facial Surgeon, Geneva, Switzerland

Arthur Swift MD
The Westmount Institute of Plastic Surgery, Montreal, QC, Canada

Jeff Watson MD
Moradi M.D., Vista, CA, USA

Woffles T.L. Wu MBBS, FRCS(Edin), FAMS (Plastic Surg)
Woffles Wu Aesthetic Surgery and Laser Centre, Singapore

Foreword

It gives us great pleasure to introduce *Injectable Fillers: Facial Contouring and Shaping*, edited by our esteemed colleagues, Drs. Jones and Swift. To say this book is timely would be understating the significance of its content. The last decade has deepened our understanding of anatomy and the effects of ageing in the face. We know, for example, that volume loss within the soft tissues combines with bony remodelling to effect significant changes, and we recognize the way that these changes are intricately linked. In turn, this knowledge has refined our techniques and the products we use to produce optimal results – a paradigm shift from the two-dimensional filling of lines and folds to a full-face approach in which augmentation begins with the restoration of the underlying structure and support that has been lost over time. It is no longer possible to treat one area in isolation without considering the picture as a whole. We have become artists with a deep appreciation of the human face in all its symmetry and harmony.

With so many advances in so few years, keeping up to date has never been more important. *Injectable Fillers: Facial Contouring and Shaping* synthesizes the most current information and state-of-the-art injection practices from skilled clinicians across the globe. The authors represent a broad cross-section of acknowledged experts within the fields of cosmetic dermatology and plastic surgery.

Dr. Jones is a world-renowned leader in the field of minimally invasive facial aesthetics. With numerous peer-reviewed publications and book chapters, he knows everything there is to know about injectable fillers and has participated as a key investigator for some of today's leading products in facial rejuvenation. Dr. Swift is an eminent plastic surgeon with over 30 years' experience in shaping and contouring the face and body. He has been recognized for his contributions for the advancement of aesthetic medicine and rewarded for his innovations in teaching and clinical practice.

As editors of *Injectable Fillers: Facial Contouring and Shaping*, Drs. Jones and Swift have created an indispensable book for the busy cosmetic practitioner who wishes to refine his or her techniques in the art of creating beautiful faces.

Jean Carruthers
Alastair Carruthers
Vancouver, 2018

About the Companion Website

This book is accompanied by a companion website:

www.wiley.com/go/jones/injectable_fillers

The website includes:
• Videos

Scan this QR code to visit the companion website:

CHAPTER 1

Injection Anatomy: Avoiding the Disastrous Complication

Arthur Swift[1], Claudio DeLorenzi[2], and Krishnan M. Kapoor[3,4]

[1] The Westmount Institute of Plastic Surgery, Montreal, QC, Canada
[2] The DeLorenzi Clinic, Kitchener, Ontario, Canada
[3] Fortis Hospital, Mohali, Punjab, India
[4] Anticlock Clinic, Chandigarh, India

Over the past two decades, neuromodulators and 'dermal' fillers have provided cosmetic physicians with the tools necessary to enhance facial features non-surgically and usually with minimal discomfort. Having a profound impact on beauty is no longer limited to a surgeon's knife wielded by an experienced specialist proficient in facial anatomy and aesthetics. Originally intended for the safer location of intradermal deposition, synthetic filler therapy has been extended beyond the eradication of unwanted wrinkles and folds into the realm of facial contouring and volume restoration. The transition of more robust fillers into deeper treatment planes by practitioners unfamiliar with the attendant vital anatomy has resulted in the appearance of devastating intravascular complications.

Complications have arisen from the use of various dermal fillers since their inception. Historically, paraffin, Vaseline, and many other materials were used that could not only cause many of the same types of devastating vascular complications, but also result in serious adverse events that were long lasting due to tissue incompatibility and immune-mediated issues [1]. Fat may be considered the archetype of 'deep' fillers, and embolic phenomena have been reported from many sites over the decades since it was first developed as a technique for volume replacement (including blindness, stroke, and tissue necrosis) [2]. Since the development of the hypodermic needle, many different drugs that were either partially insoluble or that had serious inflammatory effects on the linings of blood vessels (particularly arterial wall linings), were implicated in many serious adverse events resulting from the ensuing ischemia when accidental intra-arterial injection

Injectable Fillers: Facial Shaping and Contouring, Second Edition.
Edited by Derek H. Jones and Arthur Swift.
© 2019 John Wiley & Sons Ltd. Published 2019 by John Wiley & Sons Ltd.
Companion website: www.wiley.com/go/jones/injectable_fillers

caused inflammatory desquamation of the arterial lining tissue. From this historical perspective, then, the present state of filler complications does not present anything new, but rather mirrors experiences with other filler materials. The most successful modern fillers (the class of hyaluronic acid derivatives) now mainly show improved results for tissue integration and also lack inflammatory effects [3].

It is imperative that all injection specialists have an intimate understanding of facial anatomy and its relationship with injection therapy so that serious adverse events are minimized. A 100% foolproof method of facial injection therapy is impossible because of the variability in facial anatomy. Anatomy textbooks only give an average depiction of what exists *in vivo*, with numerous classifications and variations of vascular patterns reported (with their intendant percentages) for every facial region [4]. It is therefore crucial that treating physicians familiarizes themselves with the different techniques available to limit intravascular compromise (Table 1.1).

Table 1.1 Techniques to limit intravascular injection.

1. Know your injection anatomy – avoid danger areas and depths.
2. Aspiration before injection in higher risk areas [5]. This is not a guarantee of extravascular location as false negatives are high. Nonetheless, it is still the authors' recommendation, especially in higher risk areas.
3. Slow injections with the least amount of pressure [6] (definitely advantageous). Adverse events will commonly occur when the injector is rushing to complete a treatment.
4. Move the tip of the needle slightly with delivery of the product [7]. Although theoretically this will limit the amount of possible embolic material, it is controversial as the tip can move in or move out of a vessel.
5. Incremental injections of 0.1–0.2 cm^3 of product [8]. Severe adverse events have been associated with a significant deposition of product.
6. Small syringe to deliver precise aliquots [9]. The amount of product deposited over time is a significant factor in embolic events.
7. Small needles to slow the injection speed [10]. This is controversial in that the higher gauge can conversely access the smaller diameter vessels inaccessible to larger bore needles.
8. Blunt flexible microcannulae [11]. Intravascular transgression is still possible and has been reported. A cavalier approach is not warranted.
9. Addition of a small amount of vasoconstrictor in the product or as a preparatory step may effect some vasoconstriction without the long lasting block nor blanching of the skin [12].
10. Patient selection (e.g. previous surgery with scarred beds portends an increased risk of a vascular event).
11. The injector should always observe the skin at the area of injection and not the syringe in his/her hand, just as a driver watches the road and not the steering wheel. Drivers have rear view mirrors into which they glance to prevent accidents – so too does the injector whose rear view mirror is the glabellar region. Glabellar blanching can be the first indication of intravascular injection in the face regardless of the injection location. Therefore occasional glancing into the 'rear view mirror' of the glabellar region for signs of blanching, *regardless of the site of facial injection*, is advisable.
12. The occurrence of patient pain distant to the site of injection, in spite of lidocaine with the commercially available products [13]. (N.B. This is not noted in every case)
13. The possibility of delayed onset (several hours later) of symptoms and signs that require emergent care [14].

In principle, all the facial areas currently considered for treatment can be divided into higher risk or lower risk areas, but as we shall see, there are no 'zero risk' areas. This is an important detail that is often glossed over by manufacturers, who are keen to promote fillers as safe and effective. As the numbers of practitioners (who often learn the techniques in a weekend course) increase, certain trends in complications have been identified. One important issue is that many new practitioners have no recent experience with the vascular anatomy of the face, and worse, are completely unfamiliar with the previous reports of serious complications with the use of fillers. The combination of exuberance for a new technique, its seemingly easy implementation, and the lack of knowledge of the consequences of severe complications, has resulted in many unrecognized adverse events with high morbidity. Although serious adverse events can happen even in the hands of the most experienced injectors, when these are properly recognized and treated appropriately, the outcome can be good, but when they are not, the outcome can be seriously debilitating or mutilating. The purpose of this chapter is to familiarize the injector with the 'injection anatomy' of the face, so that practitioners can properly gauge the level of risk for the intended treatment.

1.1 Injection Anatomy Defined

Many different categories of human anatomy have been described, most of which relate to the instrument being used and the ensuing treatment or therapy (e.g. surgical anatomy, radiological anatomy, etc.).

Injection anatomy, not previously described, is centred on the use of a syringe and needle rather than a scalpel. Where the tip of the needle resides (the point from which the product will flow) once under the skin is crucial. Injecting under the skin involves encountering vital structures. Knowledge of injection anatomy therefore pertains to the *depth* of injection as it relates to the location of the tip of the needle.

Injection anatomy can be defined as the study of regional anatomy as it relates to surface landmarks and the underlying *depth* of targeted tissue and vital structures. Although a myriad of vascular patterns exist in two dimensions, there is relative consistency in the depth (third dimension) at which vessels pass through the tissues in specific geographical regions of the face. Appreciating the depth location of the tip of the needle, although not infallible, should guide treatment into 'safer' lower risk zones for specific facial regions. The clinician's ability to delineate these facial anatomical zones at the time of treatment is limited to visual and palpable topographical assessment. To this end, five bony and three soft tissue landmarks must be discerned, which divide the face into specific treatment regions according to depth (Figure 1.1).

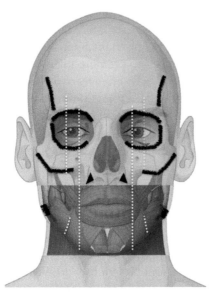

Figure 1.1 Eight topographical landmarks for defining injection zones. The five boney markers are the temporal crest, the orbital rim, the inferior maxillary border, the pyriform fossa, and the gonial angle. The three soft tissue landmarks are the medial iris, the lateral iris, and the anterior border of the masseter.

1.2 Pathogenesis of Vascular Obstruction

Intravascular deposition (either arterial or venous) of filler product, and subsequent embolization is a necessary feature of vascular compromise in the face. Unlike the distal limbs where compartment syndromes may occur from external compression, this is not the case for the facial partitions, especially considering the amount of product being deployed and the extensive collateral vascular arborization.

In terms of general organization, the arterial blood flow is from larger bore to smaller vessels, whereas the reverse is true in the venous system (smaller veins connect to larger diameter veins). Intravenous injection of sclerosing drugs works because the material is rapidly diluted and mixed with blood as the material flows through ever-larger vessels on the way to the right heart. Any foreign material in the venous system is ultimately filtered out in the pulmonary arterial system. When relatively large amounts of foreign material are injected intravenously, serious pulmonary complications have been reported [15]. However, with the small aliquots of hyaluronic acid (HA) filler typically injected, the resulting pulmonary lesions often go unnoticed or undiagnosed.

Tissue necrosis following a filler treatment is invariably due to inadvertent intra-arterial embolization of filler material as confirmed by the finding of intraluminal filler material on pathological examination of necrotic skin [16]. The filler may enter the vessel directly, as a result of intra-arterial needle tip location, or indirectly, through tissue channels created by the passing of a needle or cannula through the vessel (discussed in detail below). The embolism may be anterograde, i.e. distal or downstream from the site of injection, or even retrograde, contrary to the normal direction of blood flow (vide infra). Although filler material has been identified in the lumen of arteries in every case examined histologically [17], there is a common misconception that external pressure on a small artery is sufficient to cause skin necrosis by limiting blood flow. This is incorrect – tissue necrosis is the sine qua non of accidental intra-arterial injection. Repeated separate laboratory studies in animals have not been able to cause tissue necrosis by external pressure alone, even when very large amounts of filler have been used to significantly increase interstitial pressure [18]. This is analogous to the situation when intravenous fluid has 'gone interstitial'. There may be tissue blanching from the pressure increase of the injectate, but unless the liquid is toxic (e.g. chemotherapeutic drugs, etc.), the pressure resolves long before any tissue necrosis occurs. Similarly, extensive experience with tissue expanders has demonstrated that skin is extraordinarily resistant to necrosis on the basis of pressure alone, unless extraordinarily severe, and/or the tissues are abnormally scarred. (Tissue manometry studies carried out decades ago on tissue expanders showed that tissues respond rapidly, first by elastic and then by plastic deformation in response to pressure, and indeed, this forms the basis for the technique of tissue expansion.) Although future information may reveal exceptions to this rule, in general, any type of tissue necrosis following a filler injection is due to inadvertent intra-arterial injection [19]. The filler may travel extraordinary distances depending on the unique vascular anatomy of the area, even crossing the midline in certain situations. Almost 100 years ago, Freudenthal [20] described necrosis of the digits from an injection in the deltoid due to arterial embolism. Understanding this phenomenon explains the dozens of cases of blindness reported due to filler injections in the face [21].

Every injection under the skin violates a vascular entity, regardless of the appearance, or not, of a drop of blood from the injection site. Skewering a vessel with the subsequent deposition of product outside its walls, in a previously non-violated, non-scarred bed, should limit any adverse event to possible bruising (once the tamponade effect of the needle is lost upon its withdrawal). Application of immediate pressure over the injection site should limit this untoward aesthetic consequence.

As mentioned earlier, intravascular instillation of product may occur as a result of the tip of the needle being located inside the vessel, or more uncommonly as a result of a side-cut in the vessel created by the needle in zones of scarring where subsequent flow of product follows the tunnel created back into the vessel. With the tip of the needle inadvertently located within a vessel, once the plunger of the syringe is depressed, the pressure generated at the tip of the needle surpasses the systolic pressure within the vascular system. The flood of product that ensues is indifferent to the actual direction of blood flow, and obeys Poisseuile's law of resistance, which is inversely related to the radius (to the fourth power) of the vessel (Figure 1.2). Initial intravascular injection, if the pressure is sufficient, proceeds in a retrograde fashion down the larger proximal vessel, and subsequent distal laminar flow down tributaries ensues once the pressure from the plunger is released [22]. The local pressure gradient of the blood inside the artery in comparison to the pressure of the product at the tip of the needle will determine the direction of flow. A slowly injected filler may gradually fill the distal artery, then fill proximal to the site of injection. From there, it may travel along collateral vessels or tributaries to distal sites. This explains the occurrence of biopsy-proven arteriolar embolization in the purple livedo reticularis skin zones proximal to the actual needle insertion site. Therefore, any complaint of even a late occurring 'bruise' remote to the site of injection necessitates that the patient is seen to rule out a possible vascular event. A very large bolus can be thus expected to completely fill the distal vessel, then fill the proximal vessel past the branch points and into the larger supplying vessels, and from there be carried to distant sites by the normal

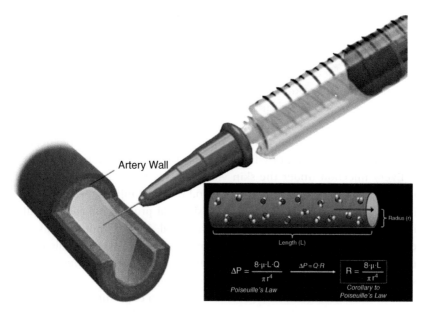

Figure 1.2 Intraluminal injection of filler results in flow of product following Poisseuille's Law preferentially down larger diameter vessels (usually proximal).

(a)   (b)

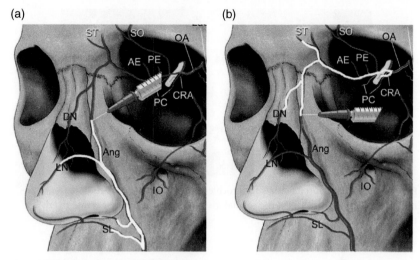

Figure 1.3 Depending on the direction of intravascular product flow, skin necrosis (a) and/or loss of vision (b) may occur.

flow of blood. The rare occasional delay in these occurrences can be explained by the initial clogging of a proximal vessel without obvious vascular compromise (due to distal collateral flow from adjacent vessels), followed hours later by dislodging of the product with resultant distal arteriolar branch obstruction (beyond the ability of collateral vessels to supply additional circulation). However, usually the effects of ischemia are immediate, with instantaneous skin blanching, followed by livedo, then dusky blue-black discoloration of the skin. Because most commercially successful fillers are now compounded with lidocaine, pain may no longer be an early sign of embolism. Fillers vary in their cohesivity, and very 'thin' fillers (reconstituted fillers in particular) may travel further into the smaller pre-capillary arterioles compared with the more viscous fillers, which become lodged in the larger arteries.

In summary, a typical vascular adverse event is due to filler material inside the arterial lumen. The filler may be propagated distal or proximal to the site of injection (Figure 1.3), and may cross the midline through collateral vessels.

1.3 The Forehead

The main arterial supply to the forehead is from three vessels: the paired supraorbital (SO) and supratrochlear (ST) vessels (internal carotid origin), and the frontal ramii of the bilateral superficial temporal arteries (external carotid origin). These latter vessels most often anastomose with the supraorbital

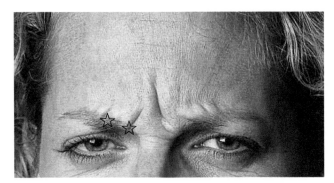

Figure 1.4 The supraorbital and supratrochlear arteries are extensions of the ophthalmic artery and exit the skull at the medial iris and medial corrugator crease overlying the supraorbital ridge, respectively.

or supratrochlear arteries, completing direct links for the entire forehead arterial supply with the ophthalmic artery within the orbit.

The SO and ST arteries (the extracranial continuations of the ophthalmic artery), exit the orbital fossa at the level of the supraorbital rim (SOR) of the frontal bone (Figure 1.4). Retrograde flow of product through these vessels allows for direct access to the globe and has been implicated in visual loss due to embolization of the central retinal artery.

The SO artery origin is typically found at the eyebrow level within 1 mm from a vertical line above the medial canthus, and is one of the most consistent anatomical findings of the upper third of the face [23]. In anywhere from 50 to 80% of anatomical dissections, it emerges through a notch that is palpable above the medial iris, 20% of the time through a foramen or ostium that is not palpable, and 20% of cases show a notch on one side and a foramen on the other [24]. The supratrochlear vessel location in the glabellar region is more variable, emerging from the orbit by coursing around the SOR 8–12 mm medial to the origin of its SO counterpart. Topographically, it can be located directly beneath or 2 mm lateral to the most medial crease of the contracted corrugator supercilii muscle.

Upon their emergence from the skull, and within 1 cm of their exit, the SO and ST arteries pierce the galea underlying the forehead muscles to ascend the forehead initially within the glabellar complex of muscles. These vessels course from deep to superficial for the next 1.5 cm as they continue within the substance of the frontalis to lie on the muscle's superficial aspect (Figure 1.5) under its anterior fascia [25]. With increased intravascular pressure and its associated vascular dilatation during exercise exertion, the pulsating arteries or accompanying engorged veins can be visualized along their superficial courses beginning approximately 1.5 cm above the

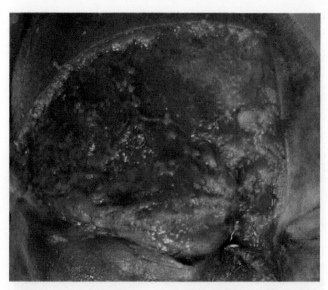

Figure 1.5 The emergence of the major vessels of the forehead on the surface of the frontalis muscle 1.5 cm above the orbital rim. The frontal branch of the superficial temporal artery can be seen anastomosing with these vessels in the forehead.

SOR. They are not apparent in the eyebrow region as the vessels lie deep within the glabellar complex of muscles (Figure 1.6). This area extending for 1.5 cm above the SOR should therefore be considered a 'no fly zone' for needle penetration below the skin. The minimal thickness of tissue from epidermis to bone in this region is approximately 2.9 mm [26]. The diameter of the SO and supratrochlear vessels can approach 1.8 mm, leaving an unmanageable margin of safety for product deposition under the skin [27].

The subgaleal/supraperiosteal plane superior to this 'needle no fly zone' remains relatively avascular, devoid of major vessels, as is evidenced by its frequent choice for bicoronal and endoscopic forehead lifts. The safer depth for filler deposition would logically be on bone of the forehead (supraperiosteal) above the 1.5 cm 'needle no fly zone' of the SOR region where vessel depth is indeterminate. In fact, because the glabellar vessels are terminal and have no collaterals, it must be stated that the entire no-fly zone should be considered a high risk area for filler injection. It should be noted that deep periosteal branches of the supratrochlear and SO arteries have been described [28], the former of which is intentionally preserved for increased circulation to forehead flaps designed for nasal reconstruction (Figure 1.7). These vessels should be of minimal consequence in supraperiosteal deposition of forehead contouring filler, as the majority of the superficial supratrochlear blood supply to the forehead skin would be unviolated, and retrograde flow of product in this deep branch is highly unlikely due to the small calibre and tortuosity of the vessel.

(a)

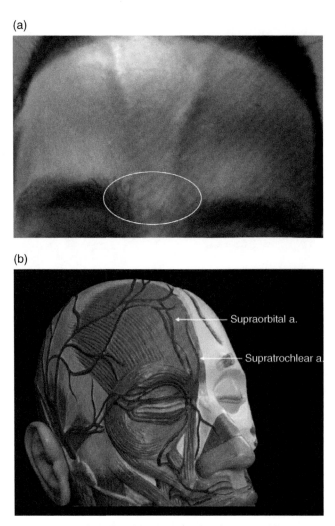

(b)

Supraorbital a.

Supratrochlear a.

Figure 1.6 Upon exiting the orbit, the supraorbital and supratrochlear arteries pierce the overlying galea at the level of the supraorbital rim. They course deep within the glabellar complex of muscles in their initial 1.5 cm (indicated by the circle in (a)) as they ascend in the forehead to lie on the muscle and under its superficial fascia (b).

The supratrochlear nerve and superficial branches of the SO nerve follow the arterial cascade in their depth and distribution. The deep branch of the SO nerve, however, remains in a supraperiosteal location as it courses up the forehead on its way to 'supply' the posterior scalp with sensation [29]. Its supraperiosteal location 1–1.5 cm medial and parallel to the temporal fusion line (TFL) deep in the forehead is relatively consistent (Figure 1.8). Nerve impingement in this region by deep needle penetration on bone is not recommended in order to avoid causing referred pain in the posterior scalp. Furthermore, several cases have come to the attention of the authors

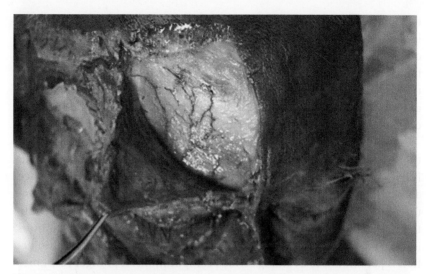

Figure 1.7 Tortuous deep periosteal branches of the supraorbital and supratrochlear arteries.

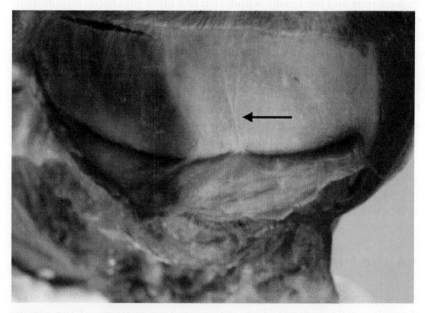

Figure 1.8 The deep branch of the supraorbital nerve (black arrow) is shown ascending the forehead on the periosteum medial to the temporal fusion line. The frontalis muscle is retracted inferiorly.

of accidental intraluminal injection of the nerve's accompanying artery, with a resultant thin vertical band of skin necrosis in the lateral forehead (S. Liew and S. Hart, personal communication). It is the authors' suggestion that depressions requiring contouring in the 1–1.5 cm zone medial to the temporal crest (where the deep branch of the artery and nerve are located) be accomplished with more medial placement on the periosteum of the forehead and subsequent 'milking' of the product more laterally into the defect. This technique of adjacent fill and milking the product to the desired location is a general principle for treating many higher risk areas, but requires detailed knowledge of the fascial boundaries, anatomical planes, and the fat compartments of the face.

When filler is injected for persistent glabellar creases after toxin therapy, the injector must be highly cognizant of the depth of the needle in that it does not pass beneath the dermis of the glabellar region. As described above, the glabellar zone is a watershed area for the communication of the internal and external carotid systems, and represents a highway into the skull with resultant visual and intracranial adverse events. Monitoring the increased plunger resistance associated with intradermal injection is paramount to avoiding serious complications. If plunger resistance is lost during treatment, it must be assumed that the needle has passed below the restrictive distension of the dermis – injection must be ceased immediately and the needle withdrawn to a more superficial intradermal location. Again, it is vital that skin vascular integrity is constantly monitored in the glabellar region due to the preponderance of end-arterial vessels in the region.

In the event that volume restoration is indicated along the curved SO brow, a lateral approach with slow antegrade injection through a larger bore cannula (25 g or greater) is recommended. Encroaching in the radix area in a vertical direction parallel to the course of the supratrochlear vessels, even with the large gauge blunt cannulas used for autologous fat, can lead to intravascular cannulization and subsequent serious injury. A more prudent approach might involve lateral approach with antegrade injection of product. In this manner, the intravascular deposition of product will be minimal in the unlikely event of vessel penetration.

1.4 The Temple

Safe correction of overly scaphoid temporal hollows can be achieved only through a solid understanding of the injection anatomy of the region (Figure 1.9). The temporal fossa is bounded superiorly by the TFL or crest, which is most palpable at the lateral brow margin. The resident temporalis muscle of mastication is firmly anchored in its superior portion to the temporal bone, as it must exert significant pull through a musculotendinous insertion on the coronoid process of the mandible. The periosteum of the forehead continues over the temporalis muscle as the *deep* temporal fascia (an obvious misnomer), and splits into two sheaths (Figure 1.10).

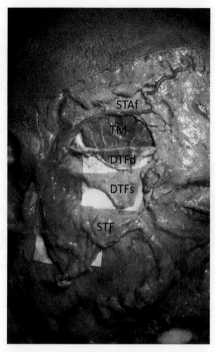

Figure 1.9 Particular anatomy of the temporal region: frontal branch of the superficial temporal artery (STAf); temporalis muscle (TM); deep layer of the deep temporal fascia (DTFd); superficial layer of the deep temporal fascia (DTFs); superficial temporal fascia (STF).

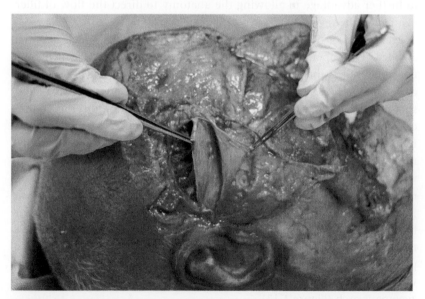

Figure 1.10 Cadaveric dissection demonstrating the two layers of the deep temporal fascia. The superficial temporal fascia containing the superficial temporal vessels is retracted to the right.

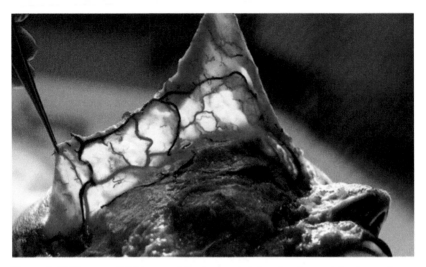

Figure 1.11 The superficial temporal fascia elevated showing the contained vascular arcade.

Similarly, the dense galea of the forehead, being unable to pass under the temporalis due to the latter's firm attachment to bone, continues on the muscle's surface over the deep temporal fascia as the superficial temporal fascia. The injection specialist can use this unusual anatomic anomaly to his/her advantage in allowing the anatomy to direct the flow of filler instilled in the region.

Every level of the temple contains vascular structures which must be avoided. The superficial temporal fascia, the deep leaves of which contain the ramii of the superficial temporal artery (Figure 1.11), lies on the deep temporal fascia. Superficial needle injection of filler in this region should be avoided, as inadvertent intravascular injection into this system of vessels can pass retrograde into the ophthalmic artery causing central retinal artery occlusion. The deep temporal arteries (anterior and posterior), branches of the second division of the internal maxillary artery, as well as the middle temporal artery, pass within the deep substance of the muscle (Figure 1.12), diminishing in diameter as they ascend the fossa [30]. The anterior deep temporal artery is located no closer than 1.8 cm from the orbital rim. A superficial plexus of veins, if not apparent through the temporal skin, can be better visualized and marked once engorged by placing the head in a forward position. The large middle temporal vein lies within the substance of the temporalis muscle 1 cm above the palpable zygomatic arch (Figure 1.13).

A single injection point *on temporal bone* is planned, 1 cm up the temporal crest and 1 cm lateral following the SOR. Digital pressure confirms the

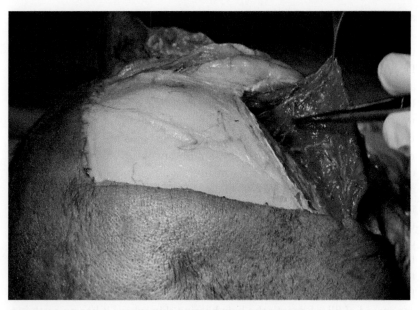

Figure 1.12 The anterior and posterior deep temporal arteries are shown on the deep surface of the temporalis muscle. The anterior deep temporal artery is located no closer than 1.8 cm to the lateral orbital rim.

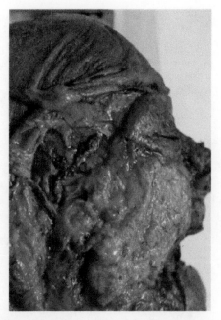

Figure 1.13 The middle temporal vein is consistently found running 1 cm above and parallel to the zygomatic arch. The transverse facial artery can be seen emerging from the parotid gland below the level of the zygomatic arch.

absence of a pulse at the injection site, and any obvious veins are avoided. A highly viscous (cohesive) or stiff (high G′) filler will ride up through the thin fibres of the temporalis muscle in this region, reaching the undersurface of the deep temporal fascia. Aspiration prior to injection is suggested, although the absence of blood reflux is not a guarantee of extravascular location of the needle tip. Maintaining the tip of the needle on bone is crucial to avoiding inadvertent intravascular injection. This location, selected high up near the temporal crest where the muscle fibres are sparse, remains relatively avascular in that any terminal branches of the more posterior deep temporal vessels are of no relative consequence to injection. The anterior deep temporal artery should not be violated as it is located 1.8 cm posterior to the crest. Slow steady injection results in subsequent spread of product which occurs in the less resistant plane between the overlying deep temporal fascia and the underlying muscle, extending circumferentially in all directions but limited medially by the fusion of the fascia at the temporal crest, and similarly inferiorly at the orbital rim. Positioning a flat finger posterior to the needle with the free hand during injection prevents the spread of filler beneath the hair-bearing skin where it has no aesthetic import. Further propagation of the filler will then result in the desirable inferolateral direction towards the arch of the zygoma (Figure 1.14). Maintaining the tip of the needle on bone is crucial to avoiding inadvertent intravascular

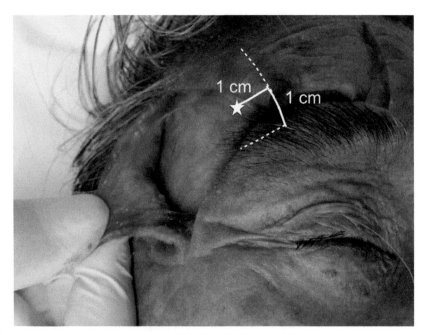

Figure 1.14 Temple injection of dyed product at the starred point (1 cm up, 1 cm over) on bone results in spread throughout the aesthetic temporal fossa.

injection. It is advisable to maintain pressure on the region for several minutes once the needle has been withdrawn, regardless of the appearance of blood at the skin's surface. This is because skewering of a deeper vessel (ex. the sentinel vein) may have occurred, and if not controlled at the time of treatment, the resultant bruising will likely appear in 24–48 hours. Inadvertent skewering of a more superficial artery or vein will result in deposition of product deep to the vessel on bone, and should limit any adverse events to possible bruising in the area. Again, in this region of the fossa, it is mandatory to be close to the TFL (1 cm lateral), anterior (1 cm superior to the SOR) and absolutely deep (the needle must be touching bone) to deposit filler in this relatively avascular plane that is devoid of any significant vessels. It cannot be overemphasized that maintaining the needle on bone during the entire *slow* injection period is fundamental for a safe outcome. It should be noted that a more inferior location for deep injection in the temple, where temporal bone is thinnest near the osseous suture line, has been associated with intracranial violation and deposition of product with a blunt cannula.

Superficial treatment of temporal hollows is also possible with the use of a lower G′ product through a blunt cannula, preferably in a direction perpendicular to the superficial temporal arterial branches. Sharp needle penetration into the deeper portion of the temporal fossa above the zygomatic arch is strictly contraindicated, due to the presence of the branches of the second portion of the internal maxillary artery in the sphenopalatine fossa, the embolization of which has led to necrosis of the ipsilateral palate.

1.5 The Middle and Lower Face

The main arterial supply to the lower 2/3 of the face is via the facial artery, a branch of the external carotid artery in the upper neck. This artery courses medially below the jaw to cross the mandible 1 cm medial (i.e. anterior) to the anterior border of the masseter muscle, where its pulsations can be easily palpated. The artery then ascends the lower face in a tortuous course towards the pyriform region of the maxilla at the nasal alar base (Figures 1.15 and 1.16). The tortuosity is understandable, as a spring-like action is necessary to allow the artery to lengthen during wide opening of the mouth. The facial vein, on the other hand, although the thickest-walled vein in the face, is more elastic than its arterial counterpart, and takes a more direct course from the central face, lying posterior to the artery and coursing through the anterior belly of the masseter muscle. Both the facial artery and vein are located deep on the buccinator muscle lining the inside of the cheek, coursing beneath the mimetic muscles risorius and zygomaticus major, and either above or below zygomaticus minor.

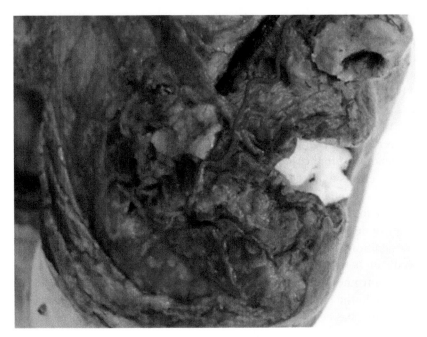

Figure 1.15 The tortuous facial artery is easily identified crossing the mandible medial to the anterior border of the masseter as it climbs towards the pyriform region of the maxilla. Occasionally, this artery may be found medial to the nasolabial fold in the pyriform fossa (see text).

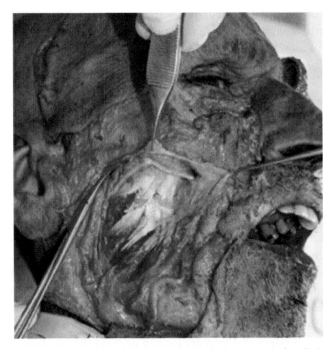

Figure 1.16 The parotid gland and Stensen's duct, which is topographically located on a line drawn from the tragal notch of the ear to 1 cm above the oral commissure. The tortuous facial artery and straight vein crossing the border of the mandible are clearly displayed.

The transverse facial artery, originating from the superficial temporal artery below the zygomatic arch, exits the upper parotid gland as the emerging artery, and divides into a superficial (superior) and deep (inferior) branch (Figure 1.13). The submalar deep branch contributes to the vascular supply of the muscles of the lower face. Therefore, injections in the submalar region, below the palpable inferior border of the maxilla, are best performed superficially in the subcutaneous plane, with either needle or cannula, to avoid encountering these deeper major vessels. Pinching out of the superficial cheek fat with injection allows the distraction of the subcutaneous tissue without drawing up the deeper vessels, adding an additional level of security. This also allows for deposition of product without violating the parotid gland or its duct (Figure 1.16).

When jawline contouring is contemplated, *superficial* introduction of the cannula 1 cm medial to the anterior border of the masseter (i.e. overlying the facial artery) has the advantage of advancing the cannula along the jawline in either direction while moving away from the underlying danger. In the authors' opinions, this can be more safely performed above the parotid fascia posteriorly. Violation of the parotid with intragland injection should be avoided to prevent untoward complications of abscess, cyst, and sinus formation or Stenson's duct obstruction. Deposition of product on the boney gonial angle may be desirable to define or re-establish the L-shaped contour of the posterior jawline which is often lost with ageing (more commonly in the female). The tip of the needle (direct approach) or cannula (indirect approach) must, in all cases, be directly opposed to and remain on the periosteum of the gonial angle during injection.

The zygomaticomalar region of the cheek receives its arterial supply from the transverse facial artery (Figure 1.13). This branch of the superficial temporal artery courses medially through the substance of the parotid gland, exiting as the superficial and deep emerging arteries. The deep emerging artery courses inferiorly to supply the muscles of the lower face, deep to the superficial zone of injection described above. The superficial emerging artery arborizes extensively over the lateral cheek, similar to the plexus of veins located in the area. Injections in this region overlying palpable bone, bounded by the lateral iris medially and the inferior border of the maxilla below, can be performed superficial or deep, appreciating the increased risk of bruising possible. Aspiration and slow injection is particularly indicated in this region due to the presence of the zygomaticotemporal and zygomaticofacial foramina, whose arteries are the terminations of the lacrimal (and thus ophthalmic) vessels. The region also houses the zygomatic ligament, a true oseo-cutaneous ligament (Figure 1.17). Deposit of filler into the deeper non-mobile fat pads (ex. SOOF) underlying the

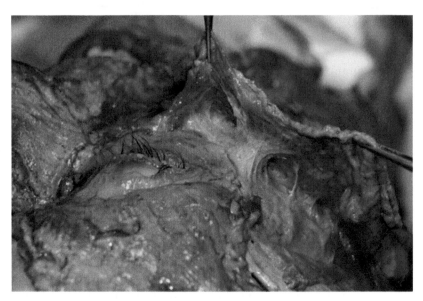

Figure 1.17 The zygomatic ligament (white) as viewed from above.

muscles of this area and pre-zygomatic space (Figure 1.18) is preferred in cases where the overlying soft tissue/skin envelope integrity is compromised (ex. the more mature patient) and unable to support the added weight of product over the long term.

The anteromedial cheek, commonly volume-deficient in the Asian population, is a high-risk area for subdermal filler due to the presence of the infraorbital artery (IOA) emerging 5–8 mm below the infraorbital rim. The artery's exit from the skull is more variable than its SO counterpart in that it can be located slightly more lateral. Often textbooks incorrectly describe it as lying on the 'mid pupillary line'. In fact, its exact location is easy to determine clinically, because the examiners finger will easily fall into the groove immediately medial to the medial border of the zygoma, about 5–8 mm below the infraorbital rim. Due to the IOA's variable depth as it supplies the overlying muscles and soft tissues, and its connections to the angular, facial and supratrochlear arteries (Figure 1.19), it is advisable to proceed with extreme caution when addressing aesthetic concerns in this region. The infraorbital foramen is angled inferiorly, commonly with a hood of bone protecting its superior margin. This exposes the artery in its foramen to deep inferior approach injections, which should be avoided. Utilization of blunt cannulas of significant gauge is highly recommended from a lateral approach while carefully monitoring patient pain and skin blanching during the procedure.

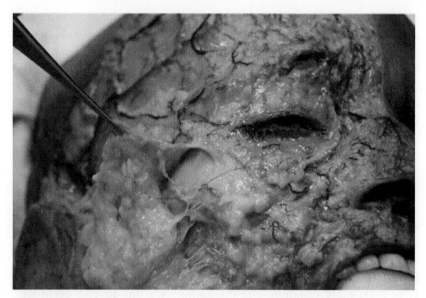

Figure 1.18 The prezygomatic space, seen here, is the preferred location for malar enhancement with fillers.

(a)   (b)

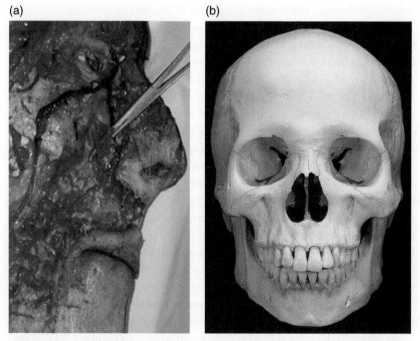

Figure 1.19 (a) The infraorbital artery is indicated and its vast communication with the surrounding vessels; (b) the angulated form of the infraorbital foramen, its overlying protective hood of bone, and the funnel like shape of the maxilla preclude an inferior approach to this region (see text).

The region of the tear trough superior to the infraorbital foramen is amenable to deep correction on the bone of the rim, although as before mentioned, this region is probably best approached lateral to the foramen, milking the product medially to the desired location. Prolonged, unresolving oedema of the infraorbital region post treatment is pathognomonic of inadvertent deposition of product behind the orbital septum, and ultimately requires hyaluronidase therapy for its resolution. Superficial subdermal 'sheeting' of filler that spreads thinly (so as to minimize the risk of Tyndall effect) may also be valuable with minimal risk of intravascular consequence.

The malar septum lies around the orbit, in the shape of a funnel, both above and below the orbit, ending deeply on the orbital margin superiorly and inferiorly, and about 5 mm lateral to the lateral canthal area on the bone. This funnel creates a potential site of complication if filler is injected superficially in this region, since it will cause premalar edema, which is just as problematic as injection deep to the orbital septum. In fact, this error is far more common, and the authors see this adverse event frequently. Treatment is again with hyaluronidase, but the problem is best avoided by injecting deep to the malar septum, and not in it. Only a tiny amount of HA filler deposited in this space (for example, a tiny droplet when withdrawing the needle) is enough to trigger the swelling.

The pyriform fossa of the maxilla, topographically located at the upper limit of the nasolabial fold and underlying the nasal alar base, is a frequent target of the injection specialist. Injections are typically placed under the alar base, medial to Ristow's space and avoiding the deep medial cheek fat compartment (Figure 1.20). Ageing of the midface is typified by retrusion of this region with splaying of the overlying alae and drooping of the nasal tip. Installation of higher G′ product as support will not only flatten the unsightly gutter, but also marginally narrow the alar base and slightly increase nasal tip projection. Unfortunately, this remains the most frequent area of intravascular injury due to the proximity of the facial artery and its frequent anastomosis to the angular artery [31]. Although most often located laterally, the subcutaneous facial/angular artery in the pyriform region (Figure 1.15) can variably course medial to the nasolabial fold in approximately 5% of Caucasians and 20% of Asians. It is therefore imperative to avoid the subcutaneous plane and place filler either intradermally for structure, or on bone for lifting effect.

Dorsal nasal enhancement is covered in more detail in Chapter 7. It is best accomplished on bone or cartilage in the midline, due to the more laterally located paired dorsal nasal arteries (Figure 1.21). Caution is paramount, especially in the radix area where the presence of an intercanthal artery within the procerus muscle can cause bruising or a more serious intravascular adverse event. Intradermal injections

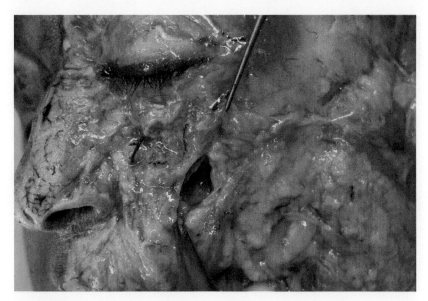

Figure 1.20 The deep medial cheek fat compartment and Ristow's space.

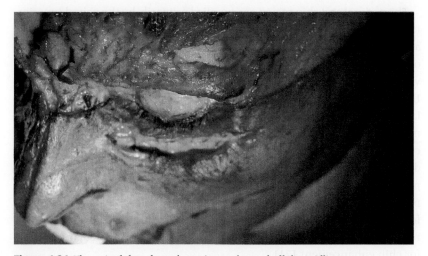

Figure 1.21 The paired dorsal nasal arteries are located off the midline.

in the nose are not advisable due to the abundance of end-arteries, the dermal occlusion of which may cause small ulcerations and skin necrosis. Every crease overlies an arterial vessel, thereby dictating off-crease puncture when nasal contouring to avoid excessive nasal swelling [32]. Deposition of filler with high G′ for the retracted columella is best performed on the nasal spine deep to the columellar artery located above the bone (Figure 1.22).

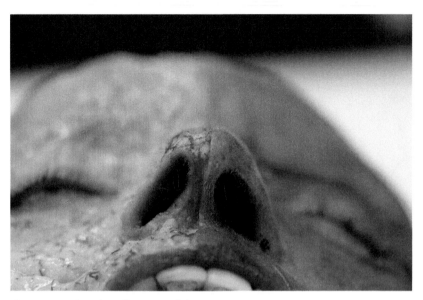

Figure 1.22 The columellar artery of the nose.

The perioral and chin region are supplied primarily by the paired superior (SLA) and inferior (ILA) labial arteries, and branches of the mental artery as it exits its foramen in the mandible. Although located most commonly opposite the first premolar of the lower dentition, the foramen is highly variable and can be found more lateral along the jawbone. The SLA and ILA are branches of the facial artery as it ascends approximately 1.5 cm lateral to the oral commissure (Figure 1.23). The very tortuous SLA has a mean external diameter of 1.8 mm and often has its origin above the labial commissure in 75% of patients. The less tortuous ILA has a mean external diameter of 1.4 mm and an origin below the labial commissure in 40% of patients. A common trunk origin for the SLA and ILA is found in 30% of patients above or below the oral commissure. The ILA can occasionally be found underlying the labiomental crease of the chin, thus explaining the reported case of blindness as a result of inadvertent intravascular injection for chin enhancement [21].

The lower lip blood supply is often augmented by the presence of the horizontal and vertical labial arteries originating from the facial artery, as well as the mental artery, thereby explaining the reduced incidence of clinically observed lower lip vascular injury (Figure 1.24). The SLA and ILA run on the undersurface of the lips both submucosally and intramuscularly. The vessels appear like dolphins, darting in and out of the muscle to anastomose with the opposite artery in the midline, but always no deeper than 4 mm beneath the vermilion at the level of its border with the white lip. Perioral rhytids and lip enhancement injections are therefore

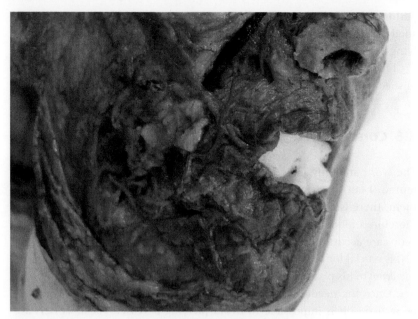

Figure 1.23 The superior and inferior labial arteries. Note that the inferior labial artery can be located quite low under the labiomental crease of the chin.

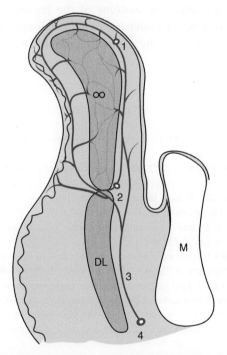

Figure 1.24 The lower lip arterial supply. 1. Inferior labial artery. 2. Horizontal labial artery. 3. Ascending vertical branch of the mental artery. 4. Mental artery.

performed with higher safety in the more superficial planes (i.e. dermal, subdermal, submucosal, and superficial intramuscular), above the underlying vessels [33].

Chin zone contouring (prejowl sulci; 3-D augmentation) can be accomplished at multiple depths, but most safely on bone in the midline.

1.6 Conclusion

The word anatomy is derived from the Greek word ana (on, upon) and temno (I cut); however, when dealing with non-surgical facial enhancement, there is obviously no cutting involved. Facial injection anatomy is therefore unique, and not typical of the 'surgical' anatomy to which surgeons are accustomed.

It is crucial for the injection specialist to have a complete appreciation of the *depth* of his needle tip in order to limit intravascular deposition of product. Once the needle penetrates the skin and disappears into the underlying tissue, it is impossible to avoid piercing a vessel. Facial vessels are extremely variable as they course and anastomose across the face from their origins to their terminal branches, but what can be fairly consistent is the depth at which they travel in defined zones.

Understanding the injection anatomy of the region and whether the needle tip resides in a vessel, above it, or below it, is critical to limiting the disastrous outcomes occasionally seen with facial fillers.

References

1. Kim, J.E. and Sykes, J.M. (2011). Hyaluronic acid fillers: history and overview. *Facial Plast. Surg.* 27: 523–528.
2. Yoshimura, K. and Coleman, S. (2015). Complications of fat grafting. *Clin. Plast. Surg.* 42: 383–388.
3. Christensen, L.H. (2009). Host tissue interaction, fate, and risks of degradable and nondegradable gel fillers. *Dermatol. Surg.* 35: 1612–1619.
4. Moretti, G., Ellis, R.A., and Mescon, H. (1959 Sep). Vascular patterns in the skin of the face. *J. Invest. Dermatol.* 33: 103–112.
5. Casabona, G. (2015 Jul). Blood aspiration test for cosmetic fillers to prevent accidental intravascular injection in the face. *Dermatol. Surg.* 41 (7): 841–847.
6. Funt, D. and Pavicic, T. (2013). Dermal fillers in aesthetics: an overview of adverse events and treatment approaches. *Clin. Cosmet. Investig. Dermatol.* 6: 295–316.
7. Sharad, J. (2012 Oct–Dec). Dermal fillers for the treatment of tear trough deformity: a review of anatomy, treatment techniques, and their outcomes. *J Cutan Aesthet Surg* 5 (4): 229–238.
8. Vedamurthy, M. and Vedamurthy, A. (2008 Jul–Dec). Dermal fillers: tips to achieve successful outcomes. *J Cutan Aesthet Surg* 1 (2): 64–67.

9. Ohrlund, A. Extrusion Force and Syringe Dimensions of Two HA Dermal Fillers. Q-Med AB, 8th Anti-aging Medicine World Congress (AMWC) Monte-Carlo, Monaco – April 8–10, 2010.

10. Lim, A.C. (2010 Feb). Hyaluronic acid filler injections with a 31-gauge insulin syringe. *Aust. J. Dermatol.* 51 (1): 74–75.

11. Fulton, J., Caperton, C., Weinkle, S. et al. (2012 Sep). Filler injections with the blunt-tip microcannula. *J. Drugs Dermatol.* 11 (9): 1098–1103.

12. Scheuer, J.F. III et al. (2017). Maximizing safety during soft-tissue filler injections. *Plast. Reconstr. Surg.* 139 (1): 50e–58e.

13. Wachter, W. Intra-Arterial Embolization with Fillers is Rare, But Severe. *Dermatology News.* June 17, 2010.

14. Bravo, BSF, De Almeida Balassiano, LK, Da Rocha, CRM et al. Delayed-type necrosis after soft-tissue augmentation with hyaluronic acid. *J. Clin. Aesthet. Dermatol.* 2015 Dec; 8(12): 42–47.

15. Jang, J.G., Hong, K.S., and Choi, E.Y. (2014 Aug). A case of nonthrombotic pulmonary embolism after facial injection of hyaluronic acid in an illegal cosmetic procedure. *Tuberc. Respir. Dis.* 77 (2): 90–93.

16. Schanz, S., Schippert, W., Ulmer, A. et al. (2002). Arterial embolization caused by injection of hyaluronic acid (Restylane). *Br. J. Dermatol.* 146: 928–929.

17. Park, T.H., Seo, S.W., Kim, J.K., and Chang, C.H. (2011). Clinical experience with hyaluronic acid-filler complications. *J. Plast. Reconstr. Aesthet. Surg.* 64: 892–896.

18. Kassir, R., Kolluru, A., and Kassir, M. (2011). Extensive necrosis after injection of hyaluronic acid filler: case report and review of the literature. *J. Cosmet. Dermatol.* 10: 224–231.

19. Cohen, J.L. (2008). Understanding, avoiding, and managing dermal filler complications. *Dermatol. Surg.* 34: S92–S93.

20. Freudenthal, W. (1924). Lokales embolisches bismogenol-Exanthem. *Arch. Derm. Syphilol.* 147: 155–160.

21. Carruthers, J.D., Fagien, S., Rohrich, R.J. et al. (2014 Dec). Blindness caused by cosmetic filler injection: a review of cause and therapy. *Plast. Reconstr. Surg.* 134 (6): 1197–1201.

22. DeLorenzi, C. (2014). Complications of injectable fillers, part 2: vascular complications. *Aesthet. Surg. J.* 34 (4): 584–600.

23. Cuzalina, A.L. and Holmes, J.D. (2005 Jan). A simple and reliable landmark for identification of the supraorbital nerve in surgery of the forehead: an in vivo anatomical study. *J. Oral Maxillofac. Surg.* 63 (1): 25–27.

24. Mishra, A., Shrestha, S., and Singh, M. (2013 Jun). Varying positions and anthropometric measurement of supraorbital and supratrochlear canal/foramen in adult human skulls. *Nepal Med. Coll. J.* 15 (2): 133–136.

25. Reece, E.M., Schaverien, M., and Rohrich, R.J. (1956-1963). The paramedian flap: a dynamic anatomical vascular study verifying safety and clinical implications. *Plast. Reconstr. Surg.* 121 (6).

26. Pejović-Milić, A., Brito, J.A., Gyorffy, J., and Chettle, D.R. (2002 Nov). Ultrasound measurements of overlying soft tissue thickness at four skeletal sites suitable for in vivo X-ray fluorescence. *Med. Phys.* 29 (11): 2687–2691.

27. Schwenn, O.K., Wustenberg, E.G., Konerding, M.A., and Hattenbach, L.O. (2005 May). Experimental percutaneous cannulation of the supraorbital arteries: implication for future therapy. *Invest Ophthalmol Vis Sci.* 46 (5): 1557–1560.

28. Cong, LY, Phothong, W, Lee, SH, et al. Topographic analysis of the supratrochlear artery and the supraorbital artery: implication for improving the safety of forehead augmentation. *Plast. Reconstr. Surg.* 2017 Mar; 139(3): 620e–627e.

29. Christensen, K.N., Lachman, N., Pawlina, W., and Baum, C.L. (2014 Dec). Cutaneous depth of the supraorbital nerve: a cadaveric anatomic study with clinical applications to dermatology. *Dermatol. Surg.* 40 (12): 1342–1348.

30. Corrêa, M.B., Wafae, G.C., Pereira, L.A. et al. (2008 Apr–Jun). Arterial branches to the temporal muscle. *Ital. J. Anat. Embryol.* 113 (2): 109–115.

31. McGuire, L.K., Hake, E.K., and Godwin, L.S. (2013). Post-filler vascular occlusion: a cautionary tale and emphasis for early intervention. *J. Drugs Dermatol. oct.* 12 (10): 1181–1183.

32. Pessa, J.E., Nguyen, H., John, G.B., and Scherer, P.E. (2014 Feb.). The Anatomical Basis for Wrinkles. *Aesthet. Surg. J.* 34 (2): 227–234.

33. Tansatit, T., Apinuntrum, P., and Phetudom, T. (2014 Dec). A typical pattern of the labial arteries with implication for lip augmentation with injectable fillers. *Aesthet. Plast. Surg.* 38 (6): 1083–1089.

CHAPTER 2

The Mathematics of Facial Beauty

Arthur Swift[1] and B. Kent Remington[2]

[1] The Westmount Institute of Plastic Surgery, Montreal, QC, Canada
[2] Remington Laser Dermatology Centre, Calgary, Canada

The Renaissance (c. 1350–1550), the 'rebirth' transition period between the Middle Ages and the modern world, has been described as the most productive era in human history. This cultural movement engulfed Europe in a revival of artistic learning based on classical sources and the development of linear perspective.

The Renaissance saw the resurgence in intellectual scientific activity, but it is perhaps best known for the monumental achievements of such artistic geniuses as Leonardo da Vinci (1452–1519) and Michelangelo Buonarroti (1475–1564) (Figure 2.1). Their influence shaped the future by empowering their generation to embrace knowledge, and stood as a testament to the development of skills in the arts. These gifted Renaissance men were more than just intellectual icons. They inspired a medieval world to break free of dogmatic ideology and endeavour to develop its capabilities as fully as possible.

Aesthetic physicians are the Renaissance artists of our time – true merchants of natural beauty and purveyors of the youthful form. Patients are our easels, their faces our canvas. We should strive to create beautiful works of art … to maximize each individual's natural facial beauty. Like our Renaissance ancestors, it is incumbent upon us to have a good understanding of the aesthetic goals necessary to achieve a beautiful and natural result, both in static repose and dynamic expression. It is essential as aesthetic experts to spend much more focused time with our patients, paying particular attention to the little changes that have resulted in a loss of their youthful appearance. Obsessive attention to detail is the key to creating great outcomes – the extraordinary from the ordinary. Our goal

Injectable Fillers: Facial Shaping and Contouring, Second Edition.
Edited by Derek H. Jones and Arthur Swift.
© 2019 John Wiley & Sons Ltd. Published 2019 by John Wiley & Sons Ltd.
Companion website: www.wiley.com/go/jones/injectable_fillers

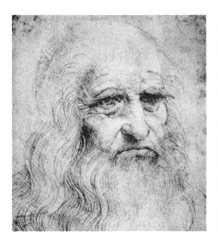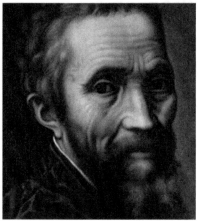

Figure 2.1 Leonardo da Vinci and Michelangelo Buonarroti.

is not to create a different look – essentially we are trying to create a form of biomimicry, mimicking what a more youthful and beautiful version of that individual should look like. This explains the necessity to study a good resolution youthful photo of the patient, to observe past balance, harmony, and proportion, or lack thereof. Very often, the most important issues are hiding in plain sight. The aesthetic specialist must be both a purveyor and a purviewer, delivering beautiful outcomes while crafting new ideas and concepts – expanding vision beyond eyesight to embrace imagination and creativity. Although certain individuals may be endowed with an innate aesthetic sense, it can be learned – at least in part – by the ardent study of art and the constant observation of facial and body proportions and relationships. There exists a sea of sameness with a flood of products, devices, and nonmedical centres, compelling aesthetic physicians to differentiate themselves through superior results. To only chase lines is a guarantee of copying the competition in a race to the bottom; cosmetic specialists must separate their clinics from the monotherapist down the street by creating exceptional results through a comprehensive global approach.

Is it unreasonable to have lofty aesthetic goals, or should we be less principled and more moderate? It would seem essential that injectors have a deep understanding and a well-cultivated taste for beauty. Otherwise they would be satisfied with a low and common goal rather than maximizing their patients' beauty potential. Michelangelo Buonarroti stated [1]: 'The greater danger for most of us lies not in setting our aim too high and falling short, but in setting our aim too low and achieving our mark'.

The world today is immersed in an expectation economy: aesthetic consumers do not want to look just good, they expect to look fantastic, immediately, and with little downtime. Patients always budget to look great because looking great never goes out of style even in a disruptive economy. Today's aesthetic patient realizes that a youthful appearance is the best thing you can wear.

2.1 BeautiPHIcation™: Optimizing Patient Experience and Outcomes

'What do women want? Women want to be beautiful'. (Valentino).

Typically, women desiring cosmetic consultation are *beauty seekers*, expressing their displeasure with unattractive ageing issues related to skin tone and texture, unsightly creases and folds, loss of smooth contours, and the presence of sagging skin. Men, however, are *youthful contenders* – their desire is to remain virile through an outwardly fresh appearance. With the prevailing culture to remain in the workplace longer, it has become important for the mature male executive to avoid the boardroom 'tired look' with its implied 'tired ideas'.

BeautiPHIcation is a non-surgical approach to restore facial balance, generate a refreshed look, and optimize beauty [2]. It treats the face as a whole rather than targeting specific lines or wrinkles. BeautiPHIcation also expands the focus of treatment beyond the desired result towards elevating the total patient experience. Purely focusing on the pot of gold denies the patient the splendour of the rainbow. It is imperative for aesthetic injectors to be both result and experience oriented. By limiting the number of punctures, the treating physician lowers the incidence of both pain and adverse events. By adopting a methodical and comprehensive approach to facial enhancement, the injection specialist can push creativity beyond rejuvenation into the realm of natural beauty maximization. Summarily stated, 'if you bruise them, you lose them; if you pain them, you won't retain them; and if you make them look weird, you will be feared'.

BeautiPHIcation uses the combination of neuromodulator and hyaluronic acid fillers to create a natural look and feel by softening deep folds, smoothing wrinkles and fine lines, restoring lost volume, and enhancing facial contours without sacrificing real expressions. The newer generation hyaluronic acids (HAs) are selected for their predictability, reliability, and reproducibility, as well as their biostimulatory and biointegrative properties [3]. Each HA's rheology defines its personality, allowing for injector artistry while maintaining complete reversibility.

This personality is related to the product's cohesivity, viscosity, lift ability, elasticity, plasticity, flexibility, degree of cross-linking, and the amount of free uncross-linked HA causing swelling [4]. The rheology determines the flow characteristics and capabilities through various syringes, needles, and cannulae. Although pharma companies distinguish their products through this scientific terminology, it must be remembered that all values relate to in vitro testing, and their relevance to actual in vivo performance (e.g. lifting capacity) may be quite different. One crucial factor, which must be considered, is the type, quality, consistency, and anatomical constraints of the tissue into which the product is being delivered. The rheology cited is best used by the injection specialist as a preliminary guide to product selection, with medical evidence-based peer review articles and personal observation then used to decide on specific fillers.

Neuromodulators based on the A strain of botulinum toxin have been firmly entrenched in the aesthetic arena armamentarium since the early 1990s. Their cosmetic use has typically targeted the wrinkles of the ageing face. As stated earlier, the goal of cosmetic enhancement is to go beyond rejuvenation into beauty maximization – creating a best version rather than a different look. Most patients fixate on eliminating unsightly lines; however, having an impact on facial beauty goes far beyond wrinkles and furrows. Maximizing attractiveness requires a comprehensive approach to restore lost volume, smooth contours, and enhance facial features naturally. Moreover, having a profound impact on beauty is not limited to the surgeon's knife. The more recent availability of 'volume' and 'structural' fillers has extended the ability of cosmetic physicians to contour facial architecture non-surgically and with minimal discomfort. Syringe therapy can create pleasing oval faces, contoured brows, youthful eyes, elegant noses, and full lips – all within ideal proportions.

In 2003, the authors presented the concept of large volume (average 15 cm³) facial contouring with commercially available hyaluronic acids (HAs) [5] by erroneously duplicating fat injection 'volumizing' techniques with the substituted HA. It has since been appreciated that large volume facial contouring remains the domain of autologous fat. The role of pharmaceutically available HA 'volume' fillers is to provide structure and *project* tissues, simulating volume replenishment. It is our contention that 1 cm³ of a firm robust HA can translate to approximately 15 cm³ of autologous fat. This backbone of the BeautiPHIcation concept was introduced in 2008 as the tent pole and canopy technique for cheek reflation [2]. Therefore, optimizing both the patient's experience and outcome requires the use of *limited, strategically placed quantities* of filler to define and enhance facial features (Figure 2.2).

The authors' concepts of facial beauty will be further expanded in this chapter as we focus on the artistic use of fillers to achieve proportion and harmony based on the mathematical golden ratio Phi.

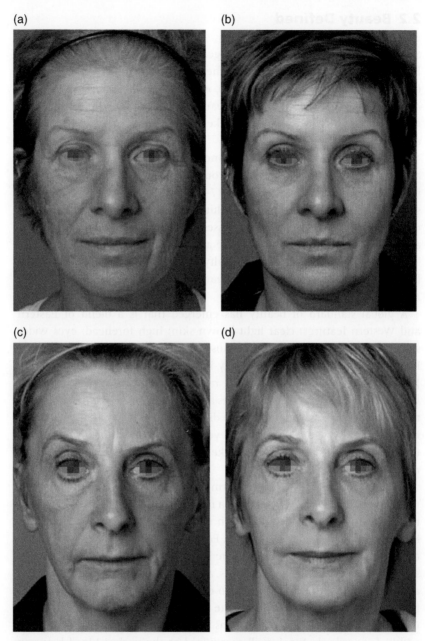

Figure 2.2 (a) Pre-treatment (c. 2011); (b) post-treatment with 4 cm³ HA; (c) pre-treatment (c. 2005); (d) post-treatment with 12 cm³ HA.

2.2 Beauty Defined

St Thomas Aquinas, known as the angelic doctor, was one of the great philosophers of the Catholic Church in the thirteenth century. He proclaimed beauty to be 'integritas, consonantia, et claritas': wholeness, proportionality, and radiance [6]. True facial beauty should arouse the senses to an emotional level of pleasure and evoke in the perceiver a high degree of attraction.

Evolutionary psychologists have concluded that humans have an innate attraction to beautiful people. Numerous studies have confirmed newborn infant preference for attractive faces [7–9]. To help ensure that our species survives and continues up the evolutionary ladder, we are genetically coded to be drawn to people who possess beautiful traits suggesting health and strong survival and reproductive abilities. Today's culture portends a beauty premium and plainness penalty – attractive individuals are more likely to be hired, promoted, and to earn higher salaries than unattractive individuals [10–13].

A global standard of beauty has emerged that is a blend of Eastern and Western features: clear light brown skin; high forehead; eyes wider set and slightly angled; aquiline nose; high cheekbones; full lips; and increased lower facial width. Beauty is universal across race and culture [14] – regardless of our ethnic or racial background, we have similar *subjective* ideas about what constitutes an attractive face. *Objective* comparators of attractiveness are much more difficult to quantify but are processed in milliseconds – we *look* with our eyes but we *see* with our brains. Does this perhaps indicate a computer-like rapid analysis of beauty based on mathematics?

The concept of a mathematical formula, relationship, or even a number that can describe facial beauty is not a modern concept. The ancient Greeks maintained that all beauty resides in mathematics. Medieval artists were impressed by the magical number 7. For them, the perfect face was neatly divisible into horizontal sevenths: the hair the top seventh, forehead two-sevenths, nose another two-sevenths, a seventh between nose and mouth, and the final seventh from mouth to chin. Novice artists are often taught that the simplest way to approximate the relative width of facial features is to divide the face into vertical fifths with each fifth being equal to 1 eye width. Leonardo da Vinci, well recognized as the perfect blend between artist and scientist, insisted that all things beautiful exhibited specific ratios known during the Renaissance as the divine proportion. Beauty is a science, 'and no human inquiry can be called science unless it pursues its path through mathematical exposition and demonstration' (Leonardo da Vinci) [15]. Many other great intellectuals, including Galileo, Michelangelo, and Einstein, also recognized that natural beauty appeared dependent on this golden ratio.

2.3 The Golden Ratio (Phi)

Used since the time of the Egyptians, the golden ratio was formulated as one of Euclid's elements, one of the most beautiful and influential works of science in the history of humankind. This ratio was known to the Greeks as the 'Golden Section' and to the Renaissance artists as the 'Divine Proportion'. The golden ratio is a mathematical ratio of 1.618 to 1, and the number 1.618 is called Phi (Φ) after the architect Phidias (fifth century BCE), commonly regarded as one of the greatest of all classical Greek sculptors. In simple algebraic terms, the golden section is the only point (hence the term divine as in single deity) dividing a line into two parts, where the smaller segment in ratio to the larger segment is the same as the larger to the entire line (Figure 2.3).

The golden ratio is commonly used today in designs and logos, and sits at the heart of the world's most beautiful automobiles. It remains one of the few mathematical relationships that are consistently and repeatedly seen in beautiful things, both living and manufactured (Figure 2.4). Ricketts [16] noted that the golden callipers applied to the human hand reveals that each of the phalanges of each finger is golden to the next in all five fingers. The broader significance of this divine ratio is that, true to da Vinci's conviction, Phi proportions govern the beautiful face (Figure 2.5). The Phi ratio defines the beautiful brow and intrinsically beautiful lips in harmonious golden relationship to the lower face.

Stephen Marquardt, a California-based oral and maxillofacial surgeon who has conducted extensive research on facial attractiveness, maintains that the evidence shows that our perception of beauty through the golden ratio is hard-wired into our 'computer' [17]. This may explain why across the world, people of different origin seem to have similar subjective ideas of what constitutes an attractive face. It may further elucidate why certain individuals lacking in seemingly striking features can still be appealing due to their near-Phi proportions. Our racial uniqueness stems from distinct diverse features and variations in skin colour, but always on a background of Phi proportioned beauty. To paraphrase Margaret Wolfe Hungerford (1855–1897), beauty may actually reside in the *Phi* [eye] of the beholder.

Youth and beauty are characterized by a full and wide mid-face narrowing to a smooth chin, commonly referred to as the 'Triangle of Youth'.

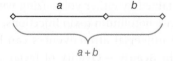

Figure 2.3 The Golden Ratio mathematically expressed. The point that divides a line into two segments where the ratio of the smaller to the larger is the same as the larger to the entire line, i.e. $\dfrac{b}{a} = \dfrac{a}{a+b}$.

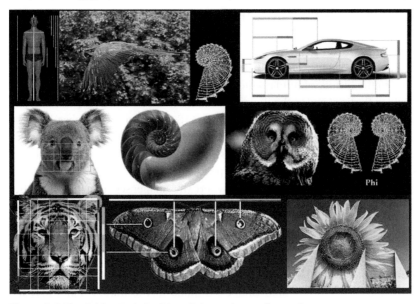

Figure 2.4 The Golden Ratio in things living and manufactured.

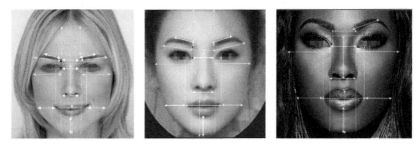

Figure 2.5 Golden ratios based on the intercanthal distance (white lines) as applied to the female face (see text), regardless of race. Setting the intercanthal distance at 1, both *Phi* (1.618 yellow line) and *phi* (0.618 red line) measurements can be found across the beautiful face.

Authoritative work on facial shape has revealed a global standard oval facial shape that is considered attractive to people of all racial backgrounds [18]. Steven Liew, a plastic surgeon from Sydney, Australia, has coined the term 'Universal Female Angle of Beauty' for the angle of inclination of the vertical ramus of the mandible [19]. This is ideally measured at 9–12° off vertical, and can be attained by either volumizing with fillers or thinning the masseter with precise botulinum toxin injections.

The components of universal attractiveness can be recalled through the mnemonic 007 Phi Beauty – **O**vality of facial shape, **O**gee curves, **7** Magnificent Features (listed in Table 2.1), and **Phi** proportions – the majority of which are amenable to injection therapy. The power of 007 Phi Beauty lies primarily in ideal proportions, exemplified by the

Table 2.1 The seven magnificent features of facial beauty.

1. Facial shape (chin, cheeks and symmetry)
2. Forehead height
3. Eyebrow shape
4. Eye size and inter-eye distance
5. Nose shape
6. Lips (length and height)
7. Skin clarity/texture/colour

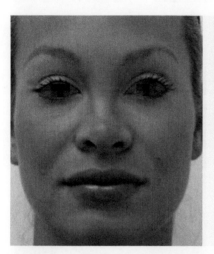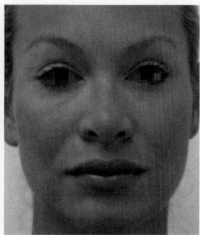

Figure 2.6 'You need volume to narrow a face'. This patient's face appears narrower after filler application to the glabellar, radix, dorsum of nose, pyriform, chin, and cheek apex (see text).

paradoxical fact that *addition of volume is often necessary to give the proportional illusion of a narrower face* (Figure 2.6).

Many papers have discussed attractiveness in terms of symmetry, balance, and harmony. Although often referred to as the 'first feature of beauty', symmetry is not absolute [20–37]. Perfect symmetry can detract away from facial beauty due to its repetitive appearance (Figure 2.7). The two sides of the face should be sisters, not twins; but the two sides of the lips should be twins with ideal proportions of upper to lower. With time, ageing, smoking, accumulated actinic damage, repetitive movements, and genetics, the phi relationships are lost causing a distracting out-of-balance appearance (Figure 2.8).

The goal of injection therapy is not limited to just restoring youth by softening ageing lines but to reestablishing fullness of features, smooth contours, and gradual transitions. Creative use of fillers will also offer the opportunity to enhance attractiveness by pursuing ideal proportions, minimizing hollows or shadows, and forming a full and suitably wide midface. Create Phi beauty, and the face appears more youthful – but trying to recreate youth does not necessarily create beauty (Figure 2.9).

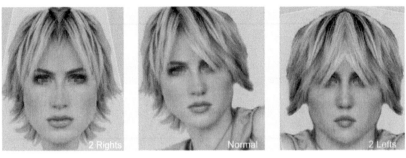

Figure 2.7 Facial symmetry (see text).

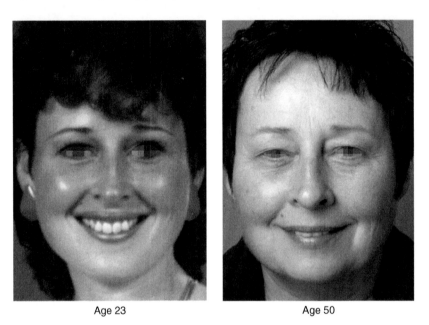

Age 23   Age 50

Figure 2.8 Changes in facial beauty with ageing (see text).

(a)   (b)   (c)

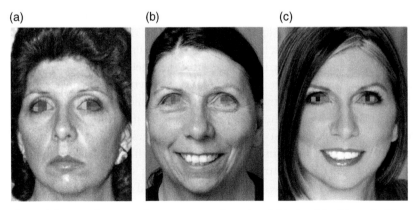

Figure 2.9 Create beauty and you create youth: patient (a) in her 20s; (b) pre-facial fillers in her 40s; (c) one month post-treatment (lifestyle photo with make-up applied).

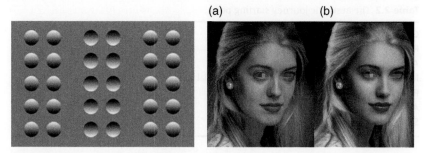

Figure 2.10 The importance of light and shadow: (a) the combination of light above and shadow below gives the illusion of projection, whereas the corollary holds true; (b) same photo with different lighting application (light above, shadow below) demonstrating the illusion of cheek projection.

2.4 Reflecting on Light

The French author Marcel Proust said, 'the real voyage of discovery consists not in seeing new landscapes, but in having new eyes'. If we look clinically with 'new eyes' at our aesthetic patients' faces and study their photos in detail, we discover that youthful faces have light and shadows all in just the right places.

Facial shadows are not simply dark areas that border the light. These shadows are as important as the light in giving life to the face. It is the facial shadows that shape the light and focus our attention to the light. Talented makeup artists understand that you cannot have shadows without light, and you cannot have facial highlights without shadows. Photography experts have taught us that photography is the language of light and shadows and that photography literally means 'writing with light'.

You must have light to see, but even with light it doesn't mean you will have 'vision'. When viewing a beautiful face, the eye focuses on areas that are highlighted with pleasing shapes. The angles that these features create are vital to the perception of beauty; highlights located too high or too low detract from attractiveness. Proper creation of higher light reflexes coupled with lower shadows can give the illusion of projection, whereas the corollary holds true (Figure 2.10).

2.5 The BeautiPHIcation Aesthetic Consult

As for all aesthetic consults, a systematic approach of recording information is mandatory. A pilot may fly hundreds of times a year, but always covers a checklist before taking off. So too, must we be methodical with aesthetic facial assessment.

Table 2.2 The aesthetic journey starting point.

Gender
Race
Age (location on the ageing curve)
Medical History (medications, allergies, previous facial surgeries, skin conditions)
Previous Injections
Aesthetic Wishes
Shape (facial outline)

The mnemonic GRAMPA'S (Table 2.2) provides a checklist of information essential to appreciating the aesthetic journey's starting point. A medical history is mandatory and should include previous aesthetic treatments (surgical and non-surgical) and current medications (especially immunosuppressants and blood thinners). Discussion should ensue of how the injectables work, how long they last, the treatment plan, the cost, the aftercare, and the possible adverse events (AEs) that may occur. The aesthetic consult seeks to create a compelling patient experience while simultaneously extracting relevant information. It is imperative to connect to and engage with your patients to understand and decipher the real reason that led to them seeking advice at this time. Also, aesthetic specialists must create serendipitous experiences, such as facial restoration beyond the patients' expectations, by addressing areas that they had not recognized as concerns.

The patient must sign a consent form outlining the risks and benefits of treatment versus doing nothing. Too little information fails to inform, while too much information may be counterproductive and only lead to confusion. Addressing the risk of blindness subsequent to facial injections has been a major concern of medical regulatory councils all over the world. The general consensus at present is for the treating physician to apply the same approach as for surgical blepharoplasty, providing the patient with an idea of the frequency of the complication in terms of proportions, rather than percentages. This is impossible to discern with non-surgical filler therapy due to the lack of precise reporting; however, from a review of the known cases of visual impairment, a frequency of around 1 in 800 000 seems appropriate. The decision of what to mention ultimately rests with the consenting doctor, but it is advisable to comment on those adverse events that exceed the 1% rule. Nonetheless, the treating physician should warn the patient of 'anything that poses a substantial risk of grave adverse consequences'. The question arises about the likelihood that same day treatment may cause unjustified duress for the patient to proceed without reasonable time to reflect on the information provided. This has led some physicians to consider areas of increased risk as a second visit procedure.

Establishing reasonable expectations before treatment ensues is a prime policy to which the injector should adhere (underpromise, overdeliver).

A particular facet of the BeautiPHIcation aesthetic consult is to educate and possibly convert the patient from the mono-focus of line-chasing to a global plan for facial enhancement. Patients' focus on lines can be partly demystified by understanding that we see ourselves almost exclusively (except in the case of identical twins) in two-dimensions through photographs, computer screens, cell phone 'selfies', mirrors, etc. Two dimensions – height and width – denote lines. Everyone else sees us in three dimensions (adding depth), implying contours, volume and shadows. Since 2008, the authors have used a brief discussion during consultation on the natural ageing process of the face, in combination with a golden-calliper-measuring tool to enlighten prospective patients as to a comprehensive facial approach. The method has resulted in conversion rates away from mono-syringe line filling to multi-syringe therapy approaching 75%, confirming our previously stated adage that 'looking good never goes out of style, even in a disruptive economy'. An added benefit is the redirection of the patient away from the anxiety of focusing on needles and the concern of pain to a stress-free discussion of proportions, mathematics, and especially beauty, thus optimizing the overall experience.

Accurate standardized photographic documentation is essential and completes the consultation process. Consistent clinical photography is invaluable in planning treatment and remains a vital aspect of the patient's record to document aesthetic accomplishments. Facial views should include frontal (anteroposterior (AP)), three-quarter, lateral, Towne view, and chin down view to highlight facial contours. Both static and dynamic views are suggested, with the patient smiling, frowning, puckering, and squinting. It is also beneficial for quadragenarian and older patients to provide earlier portrait photographs showing their youthful facial proportions and previously existing asymmetries. A useful tool is to create split face photos (e.g. age 20 and present age 50) as even the unobservant patient can quickly appreciate the need for full-face attention (Figure 2.11).

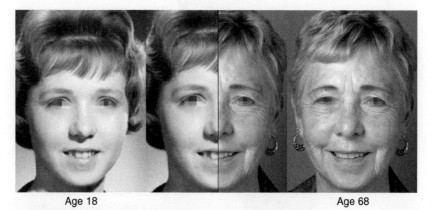

Age 18   Age 68

Figure 2.11 Split face photograph demonstrating ageing phenomena.

2.6 Changes in Beauty with Ageing

Ageing skin changes and actinic exposure lead to the appearance of lines, creases, and dyschromias. Soft tissue atrophy, with its associated volume loss, and progressive bony remodelling of the facial platform, result in deterioration, descent, and deflation (the three Ds of ageing) of the facial envelope. As ageing occurs at different rates for all parts of the face, disproportion (the fourth D of ageing) commonly ensues, depriving the face of a 'graceful' journey into maturity. A skeletonized facade results with a somewhat predictable pattern of bony resorption: the midface skeleton (particularly the maxilla including the pyriform region of the nose) regresses, the superomedial and inferolateral aspects of the orbital rim expand, and the prejowl area of the mandible resorbs (Figure 2.12).

Facial ageing is a response to the inevitable intrinsic and extrinsic stresses of life. 'Nature makes humans the same. Life makes them different' (Confucius). Not all 40-year-olds look alike. Chronological age is the actual age of a person that is listed in his passport. Biological age is the age of our cells – it tells our real age depending on how the ageing process has affected us. All living organisms experience chronological ageing, but the rate of biological ageing is 'elastic', and modulated by genes, environmental stress, and their interaction. All faces sink, sag, and wrinkle, but we do not age identically nor symmetrically (Figure 2.13). The face is one ocean with seas varying in calm and turbulence. Age-related skin changes are the

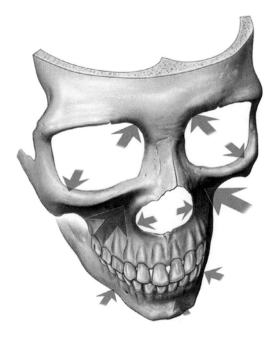

Figure 2.12 Areas of the facial skeleton that resorb in a specific and predictable manner with ageing (see text).

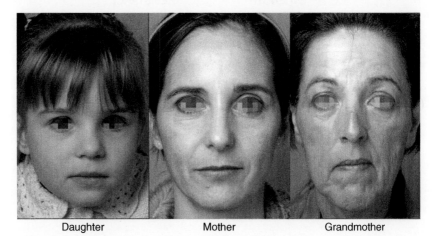

| Daughter | Mother | Grandmother |

Figure 2.13 Asymmetrical ageing through three generations. The daughter shows fullness of features with gradual transitions; the mother shows primarily periorbital and perioral ageing; the grandmother shows the added appearance of asymmetric ageing of the cheeks, forehead, and chin zone.

result of genetically programmed changes (intrinsic factors) and environmental wear-and-tear on the skin (extrinsic factors). Both influence the skin's structure and function, but extrinsic factors cause more pronounced changes through the generation of reactive oxygen species, the activation of matrix metalloproteinases, and advanced glycation end products.

The origins of unrelenting facial stress are predominantly found in ultraviolet radiation (photodamage), smoking, air pollutants (polycyclic aromatic hydrocarbons that convert quinones to reactive oxygen species), and repetitive creasing movements in areas of heightened expression. These all lead to a prototypical hierarchy of facial ageing regardless of culture or race. The periorbital region is typically the first area (third decade of life) to show signs of ageing through colour and consistency changes in the skin envelope, because it has thin skin and people blink an average of 1200 times an hour. The perioral zone, so animated through a spectrum of facial functions and expressions (talking, eating, kissing), typically shows senescent changes in the fourth decade of life. A resultant *dynamic discord* (fifth D of ageing) ensues, whereby tissue robustness declines at a faster rate than the waning strength of the underlying ageing mimetic muscles. The resulting imbalance in the tug of war between muscle strength and tissue resistance (Figure 2.14) leads to not only static imbalance (e.g. deepened nasolabial folds) but also hyperdynamic movement – wide-mouthed grins and squinty eyes when smiling (Figure 2.15), or overly pursed lips when kissing (Figure 2.16). With advancing age, this dynamic discord of muscle domination over tissue resistance creates caricatures of who we were. Neuromodulator moderation of movement in the lower face to

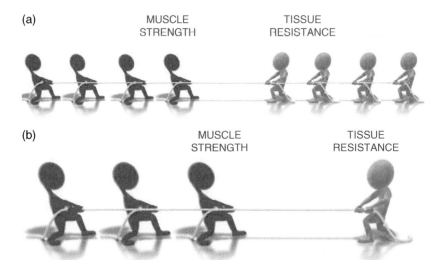

Figure 2.14 The dynamic discord 'tug-of-war': (a) youthful expressions are well balanced: (b) skin and soft tissue deterioration develop at a faster rate than muscle weakening with ageing.

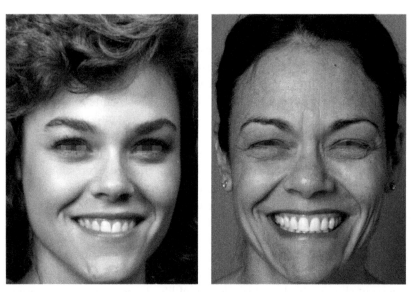

Figure 2.15 Patient demonstrating the dynamic discord of ageing when smiling causing a caricature-like facies: squinty eyes, wide-mouthed grin, deepened nasolabial folds, prominent dynamic radial cheek lines.

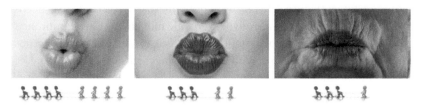

Figure 2.16 The ageing perioral region. Note the increasing dominance of the orbicularis muscle causing bunching of the lip ergotrid.

temper wide grins is extremely difficult due to the sensitivity and interplay of the perioral muscles involved. However, restoration of more natural movement is possible through the bolstering of perioral tissue resistance with structural deposition of a flexible HA filler (Figure 2.17).

Since 2003, the authors have collaborated on a global comprehensive approach to non-surgical facial beautification by optimizing facial volume and creating harmony, symmetry, and balance through reflation and contouring. To maintain natural results and avoid overinflation, individual ideal facial proportions can be attained using a golden mean calliper – a tool for dynamically measuring the phi ratio (Figure 2.18). Like the Renaissance artists who used similar callipers to determine 'divine' proportions for their compositions in stone and on canvas, cosmetic physicians can create harmony, symmetry, and balance to release the natural beauty of each individual face.

Through the changing landscape of facial ageing, the adult intercanthal distance remains constant in the absence of disease, as if a fulcrum around which the bony structures shift and rotate. Measuring the intercanthal distance in the adult face, and assigning it a numerical value of 1, a multitude of Phi (1.618) and phi (0.618) proportions can guide injection therapy to maximize results (Figure 2.5). It should be noted that basing the phi proportion measurements on the individual's intercanthal distance is a different model to Marquardt's innovative 'Golden Mask', which

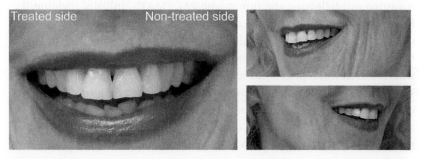

Figure 2.17 Treatment of the dynamic discord smile with hyaluronic acid bolstering of the lower cheek skin. Treatment of the right submalar radial lines resulted in a return to a natural smile as compared to the non-treated side. Note the absence of molar show on the treated side. (N.B. Photos were taken one-hour post treatment to eliminate the lidocaine effect on muscle strength.)

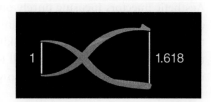

Figure 2.18 The Golden Mean calliper.

is based on the golden decagon matrix. Understanding that individual intercanthal distance does not change throughout adult life (except when involved with disease) provides the aesthetic physician with a constant measurement throughout maturity upon which reliable and reproducible therapy can be instituted. Sticking a needle into a face is easy – the expertise resides in deciding when to remove it (i.e. when the aesthetic destination has been reached). The endpoint of 'volume restoration' is not the eradication of lines, nor the bloating of facial features in an attempt to inflate sagging skin. The primary goal is a reflation process, not inflation, to create or re-establish pleasing facial proportions, reserving the softening of remaining lines and the redraping of sagging skin for other modalities (e.g. intradermal fillers, energy devices, surgery, etc.)

2.7 Facial Assessment and Treatment Planning

Consensus guidelines point to an evolving paradigm in facial rejuvenation with a shift from the two-dimensional approach (focused on correcting dynamic facial lines) to the three-dimensional approach, including loss of facial volume. The patient is examined thoroughly from all angles to appreciate facial contours, shadows, and light reflexes. Although most dermatologic diagnoses can be made in seconds, when evaluating the aesthetic face, more time, care, and patience are warranted. Systematic evaluation is carried out following the mnemonic FACEMAPS, initially dividing the **F**acial areas into vertical thirds and a periorbital region (Table 2.3). Each of these regions is assigned a value from 1 to 10 on a subjective **A**esthetic scale. There is no right or wrong value – the goal is for the treating physician to establish a priority as to which area requires the most attention. The plan is to treat the whole face, whether in one session or over several scheduled sessions, by prioritizing deficient zones. A quick but methodical assessment ensues, including **C**ontours, overlying skin **E**nvelope, **M**ovement of the region, estimated **A**mount of filler, underlying **P**latform, and safe **S**trategy.

2.8 The Upper 1/3 of the Face

Aesthetic injectors focusing purely on the presence of unsightly lines and creases often overlook the contribution of forehead and temple contour to overall beauty. A reduction in skin envelope integrity, soft tissue volume loss, and bony remodelling, all lead to an increased convexity of the upper forehead, flattening of the lower forehead/glabella and eyebrows, and temporal hollowing.

Table 2.3 FACEMAPS for facial assessment.

Facial Area	Upper 1/3[1]	Middle 1/3[2]	Lower 1/3[3]	Periorbital[4]
Aesthetic Scale	1 2 3 4 5 6 7 8 9 10	1 2 3 4 5 6 7 8 9 10	1 2 3 4 5 6 7 8 9 10	1 2 3 4 5 6 7 8 9 10
Contour (Flat; Concave; Convex; Irregular)	Forehead/Temple/ Eyebrow/Glabella	Anterior (AM)/Lateral (ZT)/ Submalar (SM)/Nose	Lips/Chin zone/ Jawline/Pyriform	Infrabrow/Lateral canthus/ Tear trough/Infraorbital crescent
Envelope	☐Thin ☐Thick ☐Average	☐Thin ☐Thick ☐Average	☐Thin ☐Thick ☐Average	☐Thin ☐Thick ☐Average
Movement	☐Lines ☐Creases ☐Furrows ☐Hyperdynamic	☐Lines ☐Creases ☐Furrows ☐Hyperdynamic	☐Lines ☐Creases ☐Furrows ☐Hyperdynamic	☐Lines ☐Creases ☐Furrows ☐Hyperdynamic
Amount (Estimate of the no. of syringes)	☐≤1 ☐2 ☐3 ☐>3	☐≤1 ☐2 ☐3 ☐>3	☐≤1 ☐2 ☐3 ☐>3	☐≤1 ☐2 ☐3 ☐>3
Platform	☐Bone ☐Soft tissue ☐Superficial ☐Deep	☐Bone ☐Soft tissue ☐Superficial ☐Deep	☐Bone ☐Soft tissue ☐Superficial ☐Deep	☐Bone ☐Soft tissue ☐Superficial ☐Deep
Strategy — Treatment:	☐BoNT-A ☐HA ☐Other ☐Intraderm ☐Subderm ☐SubQ ☐Preperiosteal	☐BoNT-A ☐HA ☐Other ☐Intraderm ☐Subderm ☐SubQ ☐Preperiosteal	☐BToNT-A ☐HA ☐Other ☐Intraderm ☐Subderm ☐SubQ ☐Preperiosteal	☐BoNT-A ☐HA ☐Other ☐Intraderm ☐Subderm ☐SubQ ☐Preperiosteal
Filler Depth:				

[1] Forehead/Temple/Supraorbital Promontory/Eyebrow; [2] Anteromedial cheek/Zygomaticotemporal cheek/Submalar region/Nose;
[3] Perioral region/Chin zone/Jawline/Lips; [4] Infrabrow region/Tear trough/Infraorbital crescent/Lateral canthus

The **beautiful female forehead** (Figure 2.19) has few (if any) lines, even tone and texture, a mild promontory of the supraorbital rim, and boasts a smooth convexity of 12–14° off of vertical that is attainable with filler therapy (Figure 2.20). Hyaluronic acid contouring of the lower forehead in the relatively avascular subgaleal plane has the added advantage of softening overlying transverse lines without the pitfalls of toxin-induced brow ptosis. Forehead height from eyebrow to hairline measures Phi of the intercanthal distance in the ideally proportioned face (Figure 2.5).

A **female temple** should be flat or slightly concave/convex, offering a more balanced and harmonious look to the upper face. An overly concave temple can detract from facial attractiveness, and signify a stigma of advancing age. Similarly, excess convexity in a female temple can portend a masculine look and distort the beautiful facial oval preferred by most cultures. Facial width should normally not exceed Phi (1.618) times the intercanthal distance for pleasing proportion. Filler therapy in this region should maintain the initial subtle concavity the temple contributes to the gentle S-shaped Ogee curve of the feminine form (Figure 2.21), and can simultaneously expose a previously hidden tail of the eyebrow.

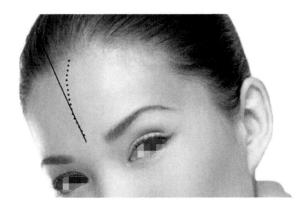

Figure 2.19 The beautiful female forehead (see text) is smooth and curved 12–14° off of vertical (see text).

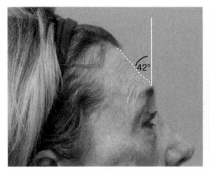 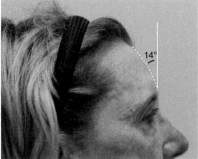

Figure 2.20 Hyaluronic acid contouring to achieve an aesthetic forehead.

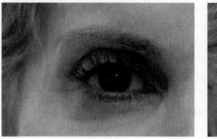 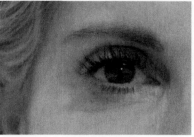

Pre-treatment   Post-treatment

Figure 2.21 Temple contouring in the female. Source: Reproduced with permission from Dr N. Solish.

Subtle differences in glabellar appearance have a profound effect on beauty and youthfulness. A **beautiful glabella** is not just about the absence of static or dynamic frown lines. Beyond the appearance of creases with age, soft tissue volume loss and bone remodelling lead to an increase in glabellar height and width, which can often be evidenced by a paradoxical elevation of the medial brow. The cautious use of pre-periosteal fillers in the region affords the opportunity to enhance glabellar beauty by optimizing the flowing curve of the brow into the radix, while maintaining the origin of the eyebrow vertically above the medial canthus at a height of 0.618 (phi) of the intercanthal distance (Figure 2.5). Further shaping of the eyebrow to Phi proportions by the addition of appropriate sub-brow volume with hyaluronic acid fillers is discussed in detail by the authors in Chapter 4.

2.9 The Middle 1/3 of the Face

The middle 1/3 of the face is the most subject to senescent deflation with ageing. Characteristically, volume 'reflation' and support as well as laser and surgical skin-tightening procedures remain the workhorses of beautification and rejuvenation in the middle face, with toxin being relegated to softening of dynamic lines or unwanted tics and grimaces. The hallmark of aesthetic filler skill resides in the central face, specifically the periorbital and nose regions, where a small difference in anatomy can lead to a big difference in appearance. Proper finesse of minute doses of filler can create more pleasing contours to the eyelid aperture or nasal profile, and impact the perception of facial width.

As mentioned earlier, the **periorbital complex** typically shows early volume depletion in the mid-30s with skin colour and consistency changes. Expansion of the inferolateral (middle age) and superomedial (advanced age) orbital rims results in a volumetric increase of the bony orbit relative to its contents. The beautiful periorbital complex is typified by richness in volume of the supraorbital brow and upper lid; even fat distribution over the entire length of the brow that obscures the supraorbital rim; and upper lid fullness that follows the natural arc of the upper lid margin. Restoration of infrabrow fullness with appropriate filler of limited swelling capacity is ideal and should not be overlooked in the mature patient (Figure 2.22).

The beautiful **lateral canthal region** is characterized by a smooth, slightly concave contour, no bony rim show, and a position 5–10° higher than the medial canthus. Filler product of intermediate firmness can be deployed on the bone of the lateral orbital rim to recreate the pleasing upward slant of the lower lid limbus (Figure 2.23).

The occasional appearance of **tear troughs** at an early age confirms the theory that they are not a true deformity but rather an uncovering of normal anatomy due to the paucity of overlying fat. This may be as a result of a genetic disposition for minimal fat in the region or of diminishing fat with age. Youthful lower lids display a smooth, single convexity rather than the 'double bubble' seen in the elderly. Volume replacement is truly the mainstay of infraorbital hollow treatment, but remains an area of trepidation for even experienced injectors due to the high incidence of post-treatment swelling and product visibility.

The authors prefer a bilayered approach to the region, using microdeposits of dilute HA both on bone and subdermally, aiming at 75–80% improvement. This allows for natural hydration of the product over the ensuing months, completing the treatment. It is imperative to avoid overfilling this

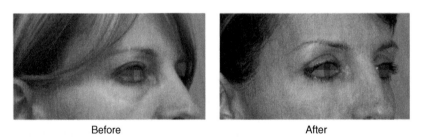

Before   After

Figure 2.22 Infrabrow treatment and brow lift with hyaluronic acid.

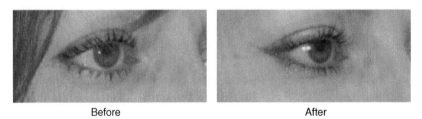

Before   After

Figure 2.23 Lateral canthal treatment improving canthal tilt with a rejuvenating effect.

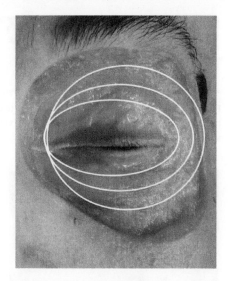

Figure 2.24 The aviator shaped orbicularis muscle is firmly adherent to bone above and below the medial canthus (coloured region). The muscle acts like a purse-string (concentric white circles) pulling the eyebrow inferomedially.

region, which will result in a distracting appearance with filler visibility during animated upward gaze. The rationale for a bilayer technique resides in the anatomy of the region, where the aviator-glasses-shaped orbicularis muscle (Figure 2.24) is firmly adherent medially to the underlying superior and inferior orbital rims. More laterally, the suborbicularis oculi fat (SOOF) inferiorly, and the retroorbicularis oculi fat (ROOF) superiorly, allow for a gliding movement of the overlying sphincteric muscle, resulting in concentric pulling towards the medial canthus with contraction. Filler injection medially on periosteum, therefore, results in deposition of product *intra*muscularly. The constant squeezing of the product with blinking and squinting milks the filler laterally where its accumulation results in a visible bluish ball (Tyndall effect). The bilayer technique addresses this particular periorbital anatomy by limiting the amount of intramuscular product susceptible to lateral migration due to the repetitive squeezing action of the orbicularis muscle. A microbolus preperiosteal technique is used for the medial tear trough followed by gentle moulding. Subsequent to this, subdermal sheeting with a cannula completes the enhancement of the region while providing a thin layer of product that hides the Tyndall of the underlying vessels. Laterally, the SOOF and ROOF provide a deep plane for *sub*muscular filler injection that remains undisturbed by the overlying muscle activity (Figure 2.25).

Nasal enhancement is one of today's most sought-after yet challenging cosmetic procedures. Although the nose is the most central and prominent facial feature, it should not be dominating in maintaining its harmonious relationship with the surrounding face. There are countless textbooks on rhinoplastic technique by world-renowned experts. It would be impossible to duplicate these refined techniques with a needle and syringe; not every

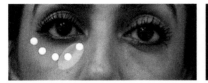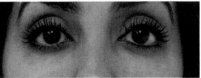

Figure 2.25 Authors' bilayer technique (see text). Note the lightening of the infraorbital skin due to the obscuring of the Tyndall vessels in the region by the thin layer of subdermal hyaluronic acid.

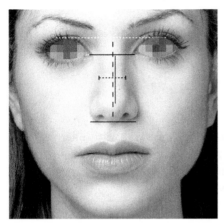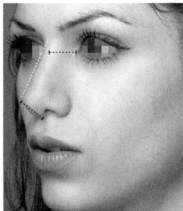

Figure 2.26 Phi proportions of the nose (see text): solid black line = 1; dashed black line = *Phi* (1.618); dotted black line = *phi* (0.618); dotted white lines indicate lashline and radix to tip line.

nose is amenable to the contouring effect of fillers within the confines of proper nasal proportion. By combining dermal fillers and neuromodulation, successful non-surgical nasal enhancement relies on the essential triad of understanding anatomy, Phi aesthetics, and injection principles.

The intrinsic beauty of the nose can be found in its Phi proportions (Figure 2.26) as well as the gentle transition between its aesthetic units. In women, the radix or root of the nose defines a nasofrontal angle of approximately 115–125°. Its projection from the medial canthus is phi of the intercanthal distance (about 15–18 mm). Its location on profile is approximately at the level of the upper lid lash line in women, the superior acceptable aesthetic limit being the tarsal fold (creating a more masculine appearance). Of particular note is a pleasing nasal length from radix lashline to columella of 1.618 the intercanthal distance; an dorsal nasal width of 0.618 of the intercanthal distance; an ideal nasal tip projection of 0.618 of the intercanthal distance; a dorsal profile 1–2 mm under a line drawn from radix to tip; a nasolabial angle of 95–110°; and two tip defining points that are the most projecting aspect on profile (Figure 2.28).

The **pyriform region** of the nose recedes with age causing nasal tip drooping, retraction of the columella and alar base widening. Nasal base width should be approximately equal to the intercanthal distance and can be narrowed slightly by the instillation of high G′ product on the bone of the pyriform fossa (Figure 2.27).

Reasonable goals in both midface rejuvenation as well as **cheek enhancement** should involve adequate volume restoration and contouring in the aesthetically appropriate locations. Beautiful feminine cheeks contain a malar mound that is ovoid, angled, and should not extend higher than the limbus of the lower eyelid (Figure 2.28). The cheek axis is not vertical but angled from the lateral commissure to the base of the ear

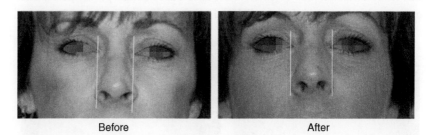

Before   After

Figure 2.27 Narrowing of the nasal base with application of hyaluronic acid on the bone of the pyriform fossa.

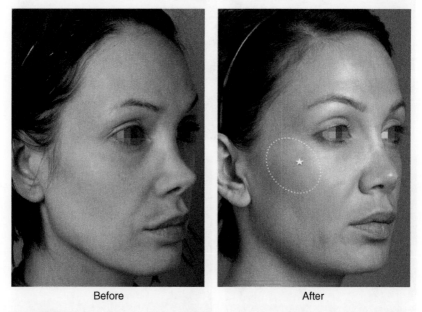

Before   After

Figure 2.28 The oval cheek created with *Phi* point defined. The patient also had temple, brow, jawline, and nasal contouring with filler. The *Phi* point (star) is located 1.618 of the intercanthal distance from the medial canthus intersecting a line drawn from the alar groove to the upper tragus.

helix. Gentle Ogee curves are desirable in both the AP and profile views. In general, ideal facial width for most ethnicities falls approximately Phi (1.618) times the intercanthal distance from the medial canthus to the ipsilateral cheek. Most importantly, each malar prominence has a defined apex, located high on the midface, below and lateral to the lateral canthus, and eccentrically located within the cheek oval. This light-relecting apex is located Phi of the intercanthal distance from the medial canthus on a line drawn from the ipsilateral alar groove to the upper tragus. The addition of a small amount of filler product at this Phi light reflex point, even in genetically full cheeks, can give the illusion of facial narrowing by triangulating the appearance. Compared with the female cheek, the male cheek has more anteromedial fullness, a broader-based malar prominence, and an apex that is more inferomedial and subtly defined (Figure 2.29).

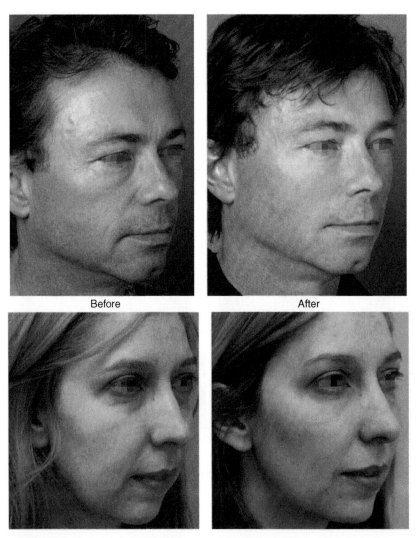

Before   After

Figure 2.29 Examples of male and female cheek enhancement.

2.10 The Lower 1/3 of the Face

The lower face remains the most challenging in the non-surgical aesthetic arena. Not only does it succumb to the loss of structure and volume with ageing, but it is fundamental to the support of the overlying senescent midface. It must not only maintain its own integrity without buckling, but must also carry the weight of the sagging cheek lying above. Furthermore, nowhere in the face is proportion more critical than its lower third. The interplay between lips, chin, bottom of the nose, jawline contour, and lower facial width is paramount to a natural, pleasing appearance (Figure 2.30), both in repose and through a spectrum of facial expressions.

The stigma of overinflated disproportioned lips has permeated the media worldwide. Injection specialists must not enable patients with poor aesthetic sense and dysmorphic requests for sausage-like lips. The art of **beautifying lips** revolves around subtle enhancement and not just pure augmentation; treatment goals should include proper proportioning of vertical height and intercommissure width (lip length), as well as recreation of a distinct upper lip white roll.

Intrinsic and extrinsic lip Phi proprotions are summarized in Figure 2.31, and can act as a template for lip enhancement. Ideal mouth width is from medial iris to medial iris, or Phi of the intercanthal distance. **Lower facial width** measured horizontally from commissure to jawline should be equal to the intercanthal distance in females, and Phi of the intercanthal distance in males. Applying Phi relationships between bicommissure lip width and lower facial width allows the accommodation of wider lips (medial pupil to

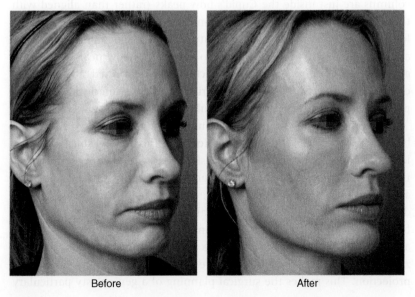

Before   After

Figure 2.30 Cheek and lower facial contouring with filler from gonial angle to the point of the chin. Synergistic effect of chin neuromodulator is present.

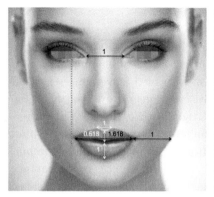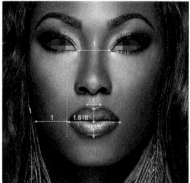

Figure 2.31 *Phi* lip proportions (see text).

medial pupil instead of medial iris to medial iris) in patients with increased lower facial width due to genetics or masseteric hypertrophy. The aesthetic upper lip has vermillion show apparent from commissure to commissure, whereas lower lip red volume is more centralized to the middle $\frac{2}{3}$ with tapering to the commissures. Upper to lower lip height ratio can vary from 1 to 1.618 in the Caucasian, to 1 : 1 in patients of colour. The lower lip should be fuller but the upper lip should project more on profile by 1–2 mm. The ratios of the distance from Cupid's bow peak to Cupid's bow peak compared with the Cupid's bow peak to the ipsilateral commissure is also 1 : 1.618. The distance between Cupid's bow peaks is phi (0.618) of the distance from the columellar base to mid-upper lip vermilion border. This is also the height of the lower lip in the midline. The upper lip philtral columns are just inside the Cupid's bow peaks (rather than aligned with them) in the youthful lip. Spreading and flattening of these columns with loss of upper lip pout is a common feature in the ageing lip. Recreation of a lower philtral column just medial to the Cupid's bow peak can restore a youthful look to an ageing lip. Injections are performed slowly, taking care to deposit very little product superiorly and more inferiorly where the philtral columns meet the vermilion tubercle.

Chin deformities are the most common bony abnormality in the face, but even experienced injectors often focus on the prejowl sulci and overlook the opportunity to simultaneously address mild forms of microgenia and volume loss in the entire perioral region. Chin zone deflation and contour changes may start early, appearing sometimes in the third decade. The advantage of non-surgical lower face contouring by adding filler volume is self-evident in its simplicity, predictability, and avoidance of the undesirable consequences of surgical intervention. The chin zone is three dimensional and must be assessed for its height, width, and projection. This makes the surgical planning of a genioplasty particulary difficult, whether by osteoplastic or alloplastic means. In many patients, inherent asymmetries in the region render these techniques incapable of properly addressing the underlying deformity. Surgical therapy often focuses purely on midchin projection and width, with no attention paid to reflation and contouring of the lateral oral commissures, mental creases, marionette zones, and pre- and post-jowl sulci. In **perioral rejuvenation**, it is not just the chin, and herein lies the distinct advantage of the physician injector skilled at percutaneous volume contouring as well as neuromodulator synergy to soften the associated apple core appearance, globally improving the entire perioral region (Figure 2.30). Historically the domain of the maxillofacial surgeon, **chin enhancement** is perfectly amenable to the physician injector using strategically placed depots of filler. However, the associated presence of severely altered dentoalveolar relationships is always better served by orthognathic surgery than by chin augmentation.

Many methods of analysis have been described to both classify and treat mild microgenia. As a general rule, anterior projection of the chin in women should be slightly behind or just at the Riedel plane, drawn tangentially through the anterior points of the upper and lower lips. In males, chin projection is preferred at least to Riedel's plane or slightly ahead of it. As stated above, golden proportions in the female dictate that an attractive lower face is described by a transcommissure distance of 1.618 in ratio to 1 for the distance from the oral commissure to the ipsilateral mandibular outline as compared to a uniform ratio in the male.

Restructuring and 'volumizing' of the chin region allows for support of the oral commissures that have turned down into the depleted marionette zones. It is the authors' opinion that the corner of the mouth in the mature patient should be neutral at rest, with a smile evoked responsively. To the contrary, a slightly persistent smile in the younger individual may seem socially appropriate.

A smooth jawline contour is paramount to the youthful appearance of the face. Understanding the interplay of the mobile facial fat compartments and the anatomical gutters created by the mimetic muscles, gives insight into the non-surgical restoration of the pleasing mandibular profile. Jowling occurs as a result of the downward and medial migration of the facial soft tissue envelope from superolateral to medial, and not as a result of pure vertical descent. This is compounded in females by the change in mandibular volume, height, and angle (the L to I phenomenon), which further stresses the prejowl tissue (Figure 2.32). Understanding the ligamentous and SMAS anatomy in the masseteric region, instillation of cohesive subcutaneous depots of HA as 'doorstops' allows the injection specialist to mildly redrape the more medial skin envelope of the mandibular contour (Figure 2.33).

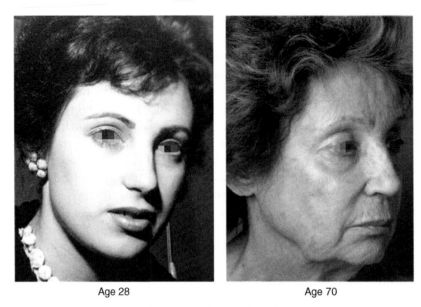

Age 28   Age 70

Figure 2.32 The ageing female mandible changes shape from an L to an I. This phenomenon, along with a superolateral to inferomedial descent of the senescent tissues of the face, leads to prominent jowl formation.

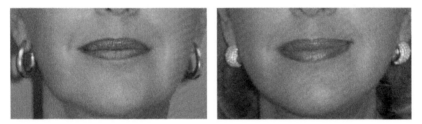

Figure 2.33 Jaw-line redraping by injection of 'doorstop' filler within the masseteric false ligaments.

2.11 Conclusion

The precise measurements during BeautiPHIcation give patients the confidence their results will be natural, individualized, optimally proportioned, reliable, consistent, and reproducible. Using an economy of product, the injection specialist can create not only a static 'best version' of self, but also one that maintains a natural appearance through dynamic expression. The doctrine of BeautiPHIcation is that it is minimally invasive, cost-effective, synergistic, and associated with minimal downtime, anxiety (for both the patient and physician), and pain. The art of bundling products with procedures – of combining fillers, neurotoxin, skin creams, and energy devices – is where technology and creativity meet.

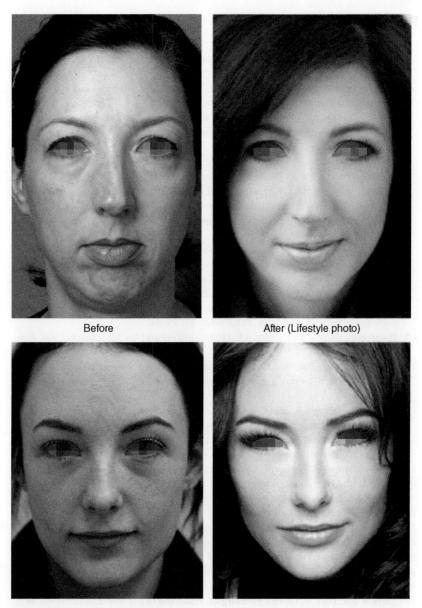

Before   After (Lifestyle photo)

Figure 2.34 Facial BeautiPHIcation.

Phi relationships can be approached for all facial features, including the nose, chin, lips, and brows. The point must be emphasized that having a plan, a facial blueprint, and using pre-treatment markings to achieve desired results are the critical element to non-surgical facial enhancement. Once goals have been determined and a budget established, a logical syntax is used to create an algorithm for selecting products and procedures. The methodology will lead to consistent and pleasing results with a high rate of patient satisfaction (Figure 2.34).

References

1. Robinson, K. (2010). *The Element: How Finding Your Passion Changes Everything*, 260. Penguin.
2. Swift, A. and Remington, K. (2011 Jul). BeautiPHIcation™: a global approach to facial beauty. *Clin. Plast. Surg.* 38 (3): 347–377.
3. Paliwal, S., Fagien, S. et al. (2014). Skin extracellular matrix stimulation following injection of a hyaluronic acid-based filler in a rat model. *Plast. Reconstr. Surg.* 134 (6): 1224–1233.
4. Edsman, K., Nord, L.I., Ohrlund, A. et al. (2012). Gel properties of hyaluronic acid fillers. *Dermatol. Surg.* 38 (7): 1170–1179.
5. Swift, A., Allergan F.A.C.E., (2003) Facial reflation. Symposium, Las Vegas, Nevada
6. Medieval Theories of Aesthetics. c. St. Thomas Aquinas. http://www.iep.utm.edu/m-aesthe/#SH3c, Internet Encyclopedia of Philosophy, A Peer-Reviewed Academic Resource (accessed 2010).
7. Slater, A., Von der Schulenburg, C., Brown, E. et al. (1998). Newborn infants prefer attractive faces. *Infant Behav. Dev.* 21: 345–354.
8. Langlois, J.H., Roggman, J.H., Casey, L.A. et al. (1987). Infant preferences for attractive faces: rudiment of a stereotype? *Dev. Psychol.* 23: 363–369.
9. Langlois, J.H., Ritter, M., Roggman, L.A. et al. (1991). Facial diversity and infant preferences for attractive faces. *Dev. Psychol.* 27: 79–84.
10. Hammermesh, D.S. and Biddle, J.E. (1994). Beauty and the labor market. *Am. Econ. Rev.* 84: 1174–1194.
11. Marlowe, C.M., Schneider, S.L., and Nelson, C.E. (1996). Gender and attractiveness biases in hiring decisions: are more experienced managers less biased? *J. Appl. Psychol.* 81: 11–21.
12. Frieze, I.H., Olson, J.E., and Good, D.C. (1990). Perceived and actual discrimination in the salaries of male and female managers. *J. Appl. Soc. Psychol.* 20: 46–67.
13. Frieze, I.H., Olson, J.E., and Russell, J. (1991). Attractiveness and income for men and women in management. *J. Appl. Soc. Psychol.* 21: 1039–1057.
14. Cunningham, M.R., Roberts, A.R., Barbee, A.P. et al. (1995). Consistency and variability in the cross-cultural perception of female physical attractiveness. *J. Pers. Soc. Psychol.* 68: 261–279.
15. Wolfram, S. (2002). *A New Kind of Science*, 859. Wolfram Media.
16. Ricketts, R.M. (1981). The Golden Divider. *J. Clin. Orthod.* Nov 15 (11): 752–759.
17. Marquardt, S.R. (2002). Dr. Stephen Marquardt on the Golden Decagon and human facial beauty. Interview by Dr. Gottlieb. *J. Clin. Orthod.* 36 (6): 339–347.
18. Goodman, G.J. (2015). The oval female facial shape – a study in beauty. *Dermatol. Surg.* 41 (12): 1375–1383.
19. Liew, S. and Dart, A. (2008). Nonsurgical reshaping of the lower face. *Aesthet. Surg. J.* 28 (3): 251–257.
20. Little, A.C., Jones, B.C., and DeBruine, L.M. (2011). Facial attractiveness: Evolutionary based research. *Philos Trans R Soc Lond B Biol Sci.* Jun 12 366 (1571): 1638–1659.
21. Langlois, J.H., Kalakanis, L., Rubenstein, A.J. et al. (2000). Maxims or myths of beauty? A meta-analytic and theoretical review. *Psychol. Bull.* 126: 390–423.
22. Møller, A.P. and Thornhill, R. (1998). Bilateral symmetry and sexual selection: a meta-analysis. *Am. Nat.* 151: 174–192.
23. Berscheid, E. and Walster, E. (1974) Physical attractiveness. In *Advances in Experimental Social Psychology* (ed. L. Berkowitz), 157–215. New York, NY: Academic Press.

24. Thornhill, R. and Gangestad, S.W. (1999). Facial attractiveness. *Trends Cogn. Sci.* 3: 452–460.
25. Grammer, K. and Thornhill, R. (1994). Human (Homo sapiens) facial attractiveness and sexual selection: the role of symmetry and averageness. *J. Comp. Psychol.* 108: 233–242.
26. Scheib, J.E., Gangestad, S.W., and Thornhill, R. (1999). Facial attractiveness, symmetry, and cues to good genes. *Proc. R. Soc. Lond. B* 266: 1913–1917.
27. Penton-Voak, I.S., Jones, B.C., Little, A.C. et al. (2001). Symmetry, sexual dimorphism in facial proportions, and male facial attractiveness. *Proc. R. Soc. Lond. B* 268: 1617–1623.
28. Jones, B.C., Little, A.C., Penton-Voak, I.S. et al. (2001). Facial symmetry and judgements of apparent health: support for a 'good genes' explanation of the attractiveness–symmetry relationship. *Evol. Hum. Behav.* 22: 417–429.
29. Mealey, L., Bridgestock, R., and Townsend, G. (1999). Symmetry and perceived facial attractiveness. *J. Pers. Soc. Psychol.* 76: 151–158.
30. Kowner, R. (1996). Facial asymmetry and attractiveness judgment in developmental perspective. *J. Exp. Psychol. Human* 22: 662–675.
31. Rhodes, G., Proffitt, F., Grady, J., and Sumich, A. (1998). Facial symmetry and the perception of beauty. *Psychonom. Bull. Rev.* 5: 659–669.
32. Perrett, D.I., Burt, D.M., Penton-Voak, I.S. et al. (1999). Symmetry and human facial attractiveness. *Evol. Hum. Behav.* 20: 295–307.
33. Little, A.C. and Jones, B.C. (2003). Evidence against perceptual bias views for symmetry preferences in human faces. *Proc. R. Soc. Lond. B* 270: 1759–1763.
34. Thornhill, R. and Gangestad, S.W. (1993). Human facial beauty: averageness, symmetry, and parasite resistance. *Hum. Nat.* 4: 237–269.
35. Langlois, J.H. and Roggman, L.A. (1990). Attractive faces are only average. *Psychol. Sci.* 1: 115–121.
36. Langlois, J.H., Roggman, L.A., and Musselman, L. (1994). What is average and what is not average about attractive faces. *Psychol. Sci.* 5: 214–220.
37. Jones, B.C., DeBruine, L.M., and Little, A.C. (2007). The role of symmetry in attraction to average faces. *Percept. Psychophys.* 69: 1273–1277.

CHAPTER 3

The Temple and Forehead

Tatjana Pavicic[1], Ardalan Minokadeh[2] and Sebastian Cotofana[2,3]

[1]Private Practice for Dermatology and Aesthetics, Munich, Germany
[2]Skin Care and Laser Physicians of Beverly Hills, Los Angeles, CA, USA
[3]Department of Medical Education, Albany Medical College, Albany, NY, USA

Loss of facial tissue volume is widely regarded as one of the most important factors contributing to the appearance of an ageing face. Changes in the facial skeleton, the contractility of facial muscles, and the stability of facial ligaments have to also be taken into account when considering rejuvenating procedures [1]. Volume restoration and facial recontouring is an essential part of modern aesthetic minimally invasive therapies using different volumizing materials. After their first approval for the correction of moderate to severe facial lines and folds, new and initially off-label indications for these agents are continually being discovered and used for volume restoration and facial reshaping.

Loss of frontal and temporal fullness is a common feature of the ageing face, often seen even at a relatively young age, resulting in a narrowing of the upper face, loss of the youthful convex frontal curve, skeletonization of the orbital rim, and a shortened and descending appearance of the eyebrow [2, 3]. While volume augmentation and recontouring in the middle and lower face has proved popular in Caucasian populations, the upper face is often neglected by both physicians and patients when planning a strategy for global volume restoration [4], with non-surgical rejuvenation in these areas mostly limited to wrinkle filling and botulinum neurotoxin injections [5]. It is important to understand that the forehead and the temple are one of the key features of the overall facial appearance, and one of the facial regions that observers first look at, due to its proximity to the eyes. A balanced approach during volumizing procedures is crucial, as a mismatch between fully volumized cheeks and a sunken forehead or temples

Injectable Fillers: Facial Shaping and Contouring, Second Edition.
Edited by Derek H. Jones and Arthur Swift.
© 2019 John Wiley & Sons Ltd. Published 2019 by John Wiley & Sons Ltd.
Companion website: www.wiley.com/go/jones/injectable_fillers

will only highlight the atrophic and aged appearance of the upper face. In Asian populations, the forehead and the temples are, together with the nose and chin, the most often requested indications for soft tissue augmentation due to the differing beauty ideals and/or facial profiles [6]. Several reports [3, 5, 7], as well as the first author's personal experience, show that smoothing the upper facial area by restoring volume to the forehead and temporal hollow, improves eyebrow positioning, and results in a tremendous aesthetic improvement and very high patient satisfaction.

The forehead, brows and temples are continuous areas and should be regarded as one aesthetic unit when orchestrating a treatment plan for the upper face. Underlying bone plays an important role in the shape of the overlying soft tissue. A recent computed tomography study of Caucasian skulls of various ages reported that upper face ageing was related to a decrease in the glabellar angle, along with flattening of the lateral orbital roof and widening of the orbit [8]. These structural changes were attributed to a visible flattening of the forehead, brow ptosis, and lateral orbital hooding. Therefore, optimal treatment results may depend on correcting deficiencies at several layers including deep structural support at the supraperiosteal level, volume repletion of the subcutaneous fat compartments, and dermal support to minimize lines and wrinkles. Recent magnetic resonance imaging (MRI) studies have also been performed that have further characterized the forehead fat pads [9].

The temple and forehead are technically more challenging to treat than other facial areas, and the rate of severe complications including tissue necrosis and blindness after volume restoration is consequently higher [10]. A thorough knowledge of the applied anatomy is therefore essential to safely perform non-surgical applications in these higher risk areas [11].

3.1 The Forehead

The youthful forehead has a gentle convex curve, when viewed laterally, with the position of the eyebrows above the superior orbital ridges and no horizontal or vertical wrinkles. With advanced age, the youthful convex contour is lost and a concavity in the suprabrow region becomes more prominent. Repetitive contractions of the frontalis muscle, altered skin collagen composition, and a reduction in superficial and deep frontal fat contribute to the development of horizontal and vertical forehead lines along with brow descent. Volume replenishment of the forehead should therefore result in brow elevation. Further improvements in the appearance of the eye area can be achieved by adding volume to the brow. An expanded brow reflects more light, eliminating shadows that can cause a hollowed appearance. The forehead is also a major determinant of a feminine or a masculine look.

3.1.1 Anatomy

The anatomic boundaries of the forehead include the eyebrows and nasal root, inferiorly, the temporal crest and the superior temporal line, laterally, and the upper hairline (if absent, the superior end of the contractile forehead) superiorly [12]. The skin of the forehead is thick when compared to the infraorbital region and contains transverse oriented septa extending from the dermis to the frontalis muscle and from the muscle to the bone. It is composed of five layers, which can be identified from superficial to deep: skin (layer 1), subcutaneous fatty tissue (layer 2), frontalis muscle and its aponeurosis (layer 3), loose areolar connective tissue (layer 4), and the periosteum (layer 5) [12, 13]. The subcutaneous fatty tissue of layer 2 of the forehead can be subdivided into three compartments: a central compartment and two lateral fat compartments on either side [14]. The loose areolar tissue of layer 4 is likewise structured by fibrous septa connecting the frontalis muscle to the periosteum covering the frontal bone. Laterally, the temporal adhesion can be identified in this layer, which is the wing point between the superior and the inferior temporal septum (Figure 3.1). Inferiorly, the inferior frontal septum separates the retro-orbicularis fat pads from the deep frontal fat pad and is laterally connected to the temporal adhesion. The supraorbital as well

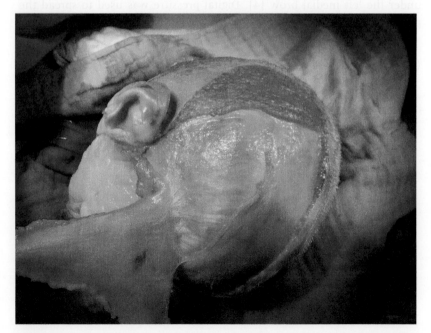

Figure 3.1 Cut edges of the superior temporal septum and stretched inferior temporal septum. Both septa join at the temporal adhesion and form the lateral boundary of the deep frontal fat compartment.

as the supratrochlear neurovascular structures emerge from the bone via their respective foramen and can be identified within 1.0–1.5 cm superior to the orbital rim within layer 4. Soon these structures change plane and can be identified in layer 3 but more frequently in layer 2, implying that layer 4 is superior to the inferior frontal septum, which is a low-risk area with limited presence of neurovascular structures in the deep forehead compartment.

3.1.2 Injection Protocol

The anatomical correlate used for recontouring the forehead is the supra-brow concavity, bordered inferiorly by the superciliary ridge of the frontal bone and superiorly by the bilateral frontal eminences. The appropriate injection plane for the forehead is layer 4, i.e. deep to the frontalis muscle (layer 3) and superficial to the periosteum (layer 5).

The most suitable fillers for the forehead are hyaluronic acid (HA) (Figures 3.2–3.4), followed by calcium hydroxylapatite (CaHA) and autologous fat. The final choice will depend on factors such as the volume of filler required, product longevity, product reversibility, number of injection sessions, and patient preference.

Carruthers and Carruthers have used a single midline insertion point to inject a viscous HA filler under the right medial brow, centrally, and then under the left medial brow [4]. Digital pressure was used to spread the product further up the forehead to soften horizontal forehead lines. The

(a)   (b)

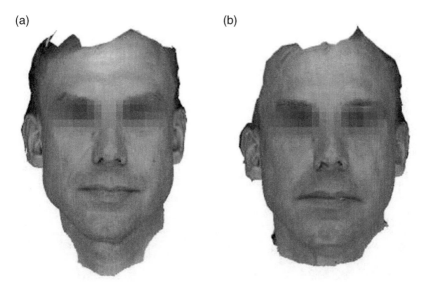

Figure 3.2 Male patient with prominent atrophy of the central portion of the forehead before (a) and after (b) treatment with a single midline injection of 0.5 ml volumizing HA based filler.

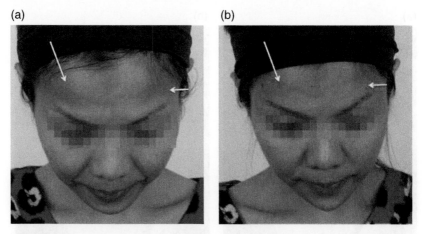

Figure 3.3 Asian woman with volume deficiency in the lateral forehead (white arrows) before (a) and after (b) injection of 1 ml of a low viscosity HA based filler.

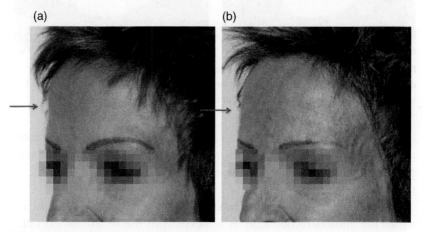

Figure 3.4 Caucasian patient with a concave frontal curve due to volume deficiency in the lateral forehead (blue arrows) before (a) and smooth convex frontal curve after (b) injection with 1 ml of a viscous HA based filler.

authors point out the importance of remaining in the correct plane, deep to the frontalis (layer 3), where it is easy to use digital pressure to spread the filler.

Busso has achieved consistent results with CaHA mixed with diluent (1.5 ml syringe of CaHA combined with 0.5 ml of 1% lidocaine and 0.5 ml normal saline) [3], which increases the malleability of the product. He injected lateral to the projected location of the supraorbital nerve in the supraperiosetal plane (layer 4) with a 27 gauge 35 mm (1.25 in.) needle, and additionally medial to the supraorbital foramen in the subcutaneous plane (layer 2) to limit potential injury to the supraorbital and supratrochlear

(a)　　　　　　　　　　　　　　　　(b)

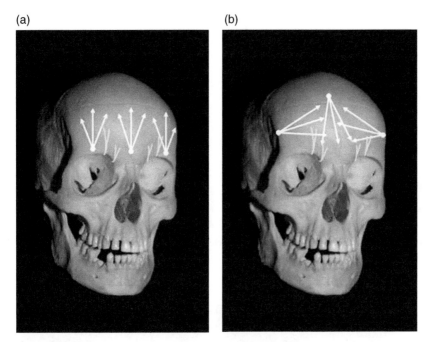

Figure 3.5 Different access points for the forehead when injecting with a blunt
cannula: (a) inferior approach; (b): superior-lateral approach. Injection plane: layer 4,
i.e. deep to the frontalis muscle and its aponeurosis.

neurovascular structures. The physician and patient should understand
that CaHA, unlike HA products, are not reversible with hyaluronidase and
that contour irregularities or other adverse events may be more difficult
to treat.

An alternative approach for treating ageing effects of the forehead,
which the authors recommend, is achieved with use of a blunt cannula,
preferably of large diameter, e.g. 22G and with limited flexibility and to
also inject deep to the frontalis muscle and its aponeurosis into the deep
forehead compartment (layer 4). Given the need to fill in a proper anatomic plane, use of a cannula is recommended given that it provides more
precise placement of filler, as compared with cannula [15].

There are two different options when choosing the access points: three
inferior points, with two lateral to the supraorbital neurovascular structures and one close to the midline with upward direction of the cannula
(Figure 3.5a), or two lateral points at the temporal crest with medial
direction of the cannula and one superior point at the midline hairline
with downward direction (Figure 3.5b).

The first author has achieved good results with the latter technique by
injecting an HA filler with good malleability characteristics into this avascular compartment (Figures 3.3 and 3.4).

3.1.3 Safety Considerations

Injury to the supraorbital and supratrochlear neurovascular structures is a potential risk when treating the forehead. The supraorbital artery, vein, and nerve exit at the supraorbital foramen, which can be palpated on the superior orbital rim, 1–3 mm medial to the mid-pupillary line. The supratrochlear artery, vein, and nerve can be found, in general, 0.8 cm medial to the supraorbital foramen [16]. As they exit, the neurovascular structures change planes (from layer 5 to layer 2) and are therefore are at risk for injury when injections are performed in proximity to the respective foramen, in the subcutaneous plane. Additionally, the frontal vein and the contributories to the angular venous system need to be respected in layer 2 of the central superficial forehead compartment. The branches of the facial artery and nerve must also be respected. These cross the zygomatic arch and enter the forehead within 2 cm of the lateral orbital rim, to enter the frontalis muscle laterally.

3.2 The Temples

Loss of volume in the temple is an early sign of ageing. Excessive concavity disrupts the smooth convex contours of the face and exposes the superior-lateral orbital ridge, the superior temporal line, and zygomatic arch, which are features associated with ageing and/or poor health. The aim when treating the hollow temple is to provide a better overall shape to the face (ideally oval) and a smooth transition from the periorbital area to the temporal hairline. A secondary effect of temple augmentation is the lengthening and lifting of the lateral brow.

3.2.1 Anatomy

The temporal region is bordered superiorly by the curved temporal crest and inferiorly by the zygomatic arch. The five-layered arrangement of the face is not valid in this area as 10 different layers can be identified here. From superficial to deep: skin (layer 1, Figure 3.6a), subcutaneous fatty tissue (layer 2, Figure 3.6b), superficial temporal fascia (layer 3, Figure 3.6c), loose areolar connective tissue and deep fatty tissue (layer 4, Figure 3.6c), superficial lamina of the deep temporal fascia (layer 5), superficial temporal fat pad (layer 6, Figure 3.6d), deep lamina of the deep temporal fascia (layer 7, Figure 3.6e), deep temporal fat pad (which is the temporal extension of the buccal fat pad, layer 8), the temporal muscle (layer 9, Figure 3.6f), and the periosteum, which is dispersed by muscle fibres inserting into the bone (layer 10). The superficial temporal artery emerges from deeper layers 1 cm anterior and 1 cm superior to the tragus and is embedded into the superficial temporal fascia (which is the

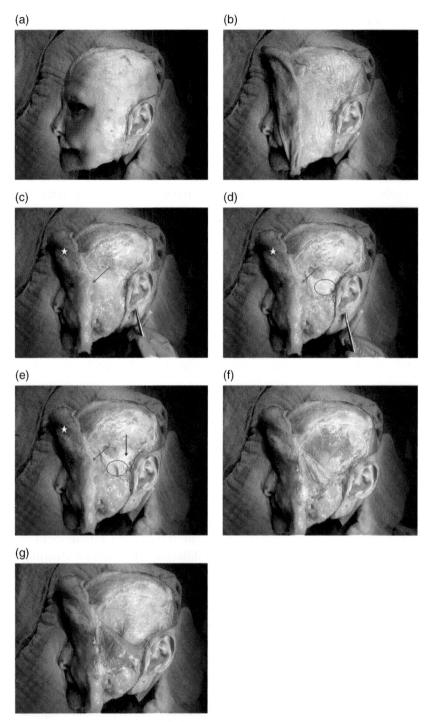

Figure 3.6 (a) Dissected head with skin of the temporal region *in situ*. (b) Dissected head after removal of the skin. The subcutaneous fatty layer is visible. (c) Dissected head after removal of skin, subcutaneous tissue, and the superficial temporal fascia.

continuation of the galea aponeurotica, layer 3) towards its course to the forehead. In the lower temporal compartment (inferior to the inferior temporal septum), motor branches of the facial nerve and sensory branches of the zygomaticotemporal nerve can be identified in the deep fat. Between the superficial and the deep lamina of the deep temporal fascia, the medial zygomaticotemporal vein (sentinel vein) can be identified within the superficial temporal fat pad. Note that between the temporalis muscle and temporal bone, a thin layer of periosteum is present that enables subperiosteal surgical procedures but this potential space is generally not accessible for minimally invasive injections (Figure 3.6g). The temporal region presents with a high variability in its bone formation and stability because the sutures of the sphenoid, the frontal, the parietal and the temporal bone have a high variability. This specific region has long been recognized as a site of minimal resistance of the neurocranium and is called the pterion. The pterion can generally be found 3 cm posterior and 3 cm superior from the lateral canthus. Another description localizes the pterion to 3 cm posterior to the frontozygomatic suture (corresponds to the lateral end of the eyebrow) and 4 cm superior to the zygomatic arch. These distances must be interpreted with great caution as the pterion can have different shapes (H, I, K, X or W shape), can vary between the left and the right side of the neurocranium, and can present with epipteric bones.

3.2.2 Injection Protocol

The addition of volumizing materials to the temporal region has been shown to restore the width of the upper face and to generate a youthful look. Treating the temporal fossa also helps with lateral brow positioning and visibility, as the tail of the brow can disappear into the hollow.

View onto the loose areolar tissue and the deep fatty layer (layer 4). The superficial temporal fascia is continuous cranially with the galea aponeurotica and inferiorly with the superficial musculo-aponeurotic system (SMAS). In this image, all are reflected rostrally as one single layer. In this layer the orbicularis oculi muscle is included (black star) as well as the frontalis muscle (white star). The temporal adhesion is marked with the blue arrow and the McGregor's patch with the red arrow. (d) Dissected head with rostral reflection of layer 3. The superficial lamina of the deep temporal fascia is flipped inferiorly and the superficial temporal fat pad is visible (red circle). (e) Dissected head with rostral reflection of layer 3. The superficial temporal fat pad is reflected inferiorly and the deep lamina of the deep temporal fascia is visible (black arrow). Anteriorly the temporalis muscle can be seen through a cut window. (f) Dissected head with inferior reflection of the deep lamina of the deep temporal fascia. The temporalis muscle is exposed. (g) The temporalis muscle is reflected inferiorly and the bony temporal fossa is exposed. To remove the muscle, sharp dissection must be performed as the muscle is strongly adherent to the bone. Remnants of the periosteum are visible.

(a)　　　　　　　　　　　　　　　　　　(b)

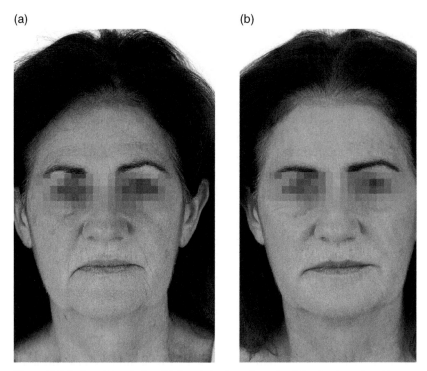

Figure 3.7 Before (a) and after (b) deep injection of a volumizing hyaluronic acid-based material bilaterally into the temple.

The authors discourage use of a needle with forehead augmentation for reasons outlined in this chapter. However, for reference, two different planes can be accessed when treating this delicate area: superficial or deep. With the former, a needle long enough to reach the bone (e.g. 25G 25.4mm (1″)) can be used to deposit boluses of a viscous HA filler, CaHA, or poly-L-lactic acid (Figure 3.7) [2, 3, 5, 17]. The needle is placed at the point of the maximal visible temporal depression perpendicular to the skin and is advanced gently until final contact with the bone is reached. With the needle tip gently touching the bone, the material is injected slowly and in small 0.1–0.2 ml boluses.

According to Breithaupt et al. injections can be performed safely in a window between the temporal fusion line (superomedial boundary), at least 2 cm above the zygomatic arch (inferior boundary) to avoid the middle temporal vein, and the hairline (posterior boundary), when applying the filler supraperiosteally. To avoid injury to the superficial temporal artery, it is recommended that it is palpated and marked prior to injection [18].

Swift has described an alternative methodology using a single injection point 1 cm superior and 1 cm lateral to the tail of the brow [19]. This injection technique is demonstrated by Derek Jones, MD, in the video that accompanies this chapter.

Recent evidence supports a high risk for intracranial penetration when using a needle to introduce filler for temple augmentation [20]. High pressure should be strictly avoided as it has been shown that forces >4 kg may increase the probability of penetrating the bone and reaching the intracranial space. As this injection technique applies the material intramuscularly, into the temporalis muscle, the patient should be asked to chew in order to improve the distribution of the product. In this plane, no major arteries or veins are expected to be found, yet great caution must be taken to minimize the risk of retrograde arterial migration, embolism, necrosis or blindness. Aspiration before injection can be a useful test to avoid intravascular injection, but it does not provide guaranteed safety. Injections into the most inferior region of the infratemporal fossa should be avoided as the product may get lost or gain access to the midface and lead to an increased appearance of the jowl deformity.

Approaching this technique with a consistent access point (e.g. 1 cm up and 1 cm laterally from the tail of the eyebrow [19]) should be performed with caution as the resistance of the underlying bone may be diminished due to the high variability of the presented anatomy of the pterion.

For superficial (subdermal) temple injections (Figure 3.8), a stiff blunt tip cannula (22G or at least 25G) is recommended. Tenting of the temporal skin separates the loosely associated subcutaneous fatty tissue (layer 2) from the superficial temporal fascia (layer 3) and accentuates the target injection space. Products that are primarily HA with lower volumizing

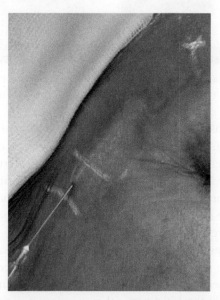

Figure 3.8 Superficial (subdermal) injection of the temporal region using a 22G blunt cannula.

(a) (b)

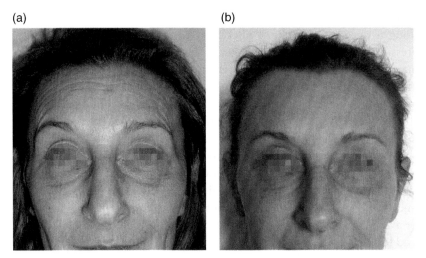

Figure 3.9 Before (a) and after (b) injection of HA fillers into the subdermal layer of the temporal region using a blunt cannula.

(a) (b)

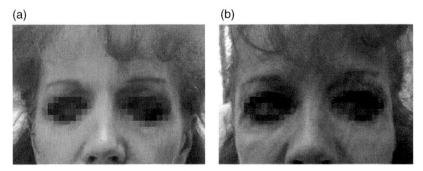

Figure 3.10 Before (a) and after (b) injection of highly diluted calcium hydroxyapatite (CaHA, 1.0 ml) into the subdermal layer of the temporal region using a blunt cannula.

capacity (low G′, high Tan δ) (Figure 3.9) or highly diluted CaHA (1 : 1) are used (Figure 3.10). Various access points can be used and of those the most frequent are: inferior (zygomatic arch), anterior (external orbital rim), or posterior (hair line). To lower the risk of infection or vessel damage, the first author prefers the inferior access point. The patient should be informed that the superficial veins in the treated area may become more prominent for several days.

Some colleagues also report success using a blunt cannula to place filler between the superficial temporal fascia and the deep lamina of the deep temporal fascia [21]. One of the crucial structures in this layer is the temporal branch of the facial nerve that may increase patient discomfort during the injection [21].

3.2.3 Safety Considerations

When applying fillers in the temporal region, the underlying anatomy and the layered concept must be considered to avoid adverse effects. The following structures are of significant interest: superficial temporal artery, middle zygomaticotemporal vein, deep temporal arteries and veins, and temporal branches of the facial nerve. While still rare, an increasing number of cases of blindness have been described following augmentation procedures to the upper face [10, 22]. Healthcare professionals should therefore always have this severe complication in mind when injecting in this area and use blunt, rather stiff cannulas (at least 25G or ideally 22G) around the superficial temporal fascia, and avoid the use of needles [23].

3.3 Conclusions

In the upper face, loss of forehead convexity and hollowing of the temples contribute significantly to an aged appearance. Volume restoration has been shown to successfully and effectively restore youthful contours to the face. Healthcare professionals have to consider the dramatic improvements in the change of a patients' facial appearance after treating the upper face as a unit and emphasize a full upper-face approach in a treatment plan.

References

1. Cotofana, S., Fratila, A.A., Schenck, T.L. et al. (2016 Jun). The anatomy of the aging face: a review. *Facial Plast. Surg.* 32 (3): 253–260.
2. Alghoul, M. and Codner, M.A. (2013). Retaining ligaments of the face: review of anatomy and clinical applications. *Aesthet. Surg. J.* 33: 769–782.
3. Busso, M. and Howell, D.J. (2010). Forehead recontouring using calcium hydroxylapatite. *Dermatol. Surg.* 36 (Suppl 3): 1910–1913.
4. Carruthers, J. and Carruthers, A. (2010). Volumizing the glabella and forehead. *Dermatol. Surg.* 36: 1905–1909.
5. Carruthers, J.D., Fagien, S., Rohrich, R.J. et al. (2014). Blindness caused by cosmetic filler injection: a review of cause and therapy. *Plast. Reconstr. Surg.* 134: 1197–1201.
6. Chen, Y., Wang, W., Li, J. et al. (2014). Fundus artery occlusion caused by cosmetic facial injections. *Chin. Med. J.* 127: 1434–1437.
7. Claude O, Trevidic P. Injection of the temporal region and eyebrow. In: *Anatomy and Volumizing Injections*, 77–104. Expert2Expert Medical Publishing, Master Collection 2. http://expert2expert.co.uk/product/anatomy-volumising-injections-mcv2
8. Lambros, V. (2011). A technique for filling the temples with highly diluted hyaluronic acid: the "dilution solution". *Aesthet. Surg. J.* 31: 89–94.
9. Cotofana, S. and Gotkin, R.H. (accepted for publication)(2017 Aug). Letter to the editor on: high resolution magnetic resonance imaging of aging upper face fat compartments. *Plast. Reconstr. Surg.* E pub.

10. Lee, S.K. and Kim, H.S. (2014). Recent trend in the choice of fillers and injection techniques in Asia: a questionnaire study based on expert opinion. *J. Drugs Dermatol.* 13: 24–31.

11. Lorenc, Z.P., Ivy, E., and Aston, S.J. (1995 Sep–Oct). Neurosensory preservation in endoscopic forehead plasty. *Aesthet. Plast. Surg.* 19 (5): 411–413.

12. Moradi, A., Shirazi, A., and Perez, V. (2011). A guide to temporal fossa augmentation with small gel particle hyaluronic acid dermal filler. *J. Drugs Dermatol.* 10: 673–676.

13. Rohrich, R.J. and Pessa, J.E. (2007). The fat compartments of the face: anatomy and clinical implications for cosmetic surgery. *Plast. Reconstr. Surg.* 119: 2219–2227.

14. Rose, A.E. and Day, D. (2013). Esthetic rejuvenation of the temple. *Clin. Plast. Surg.* 40: 77–89.

15. Pavicic, T., Konstantin, F., Erlbacher, K. et al. (2017). Precision in dermal filling: a comparison between needle and cannula when using soft tissue fillers. *J. Drugs Dermatol.* 16 (9): 866–872.

16. Ross, J.J. and Malhotra, R. (2010). Orbitofacial rejuvenation of temple hollowing with Perlane injectable filler. *Aesthet. Surg. J.* 30: 428–433.

17. Shaw, R.B. Jr., Katzel, E.B., Koltz, P.F. et al. (2011). Aging of the facial skeleton: aesthetic implications and rejuvenation strategies. *Plast. Reconstr. Surg.* 127: 374–383.

18. Breithaupt, A.D., Jones, D.H., Braz, A. et al. (2015 Dec). Anatomical basis for safe and effective volumization of the temple. *Dermatol. Surg.* 41 (Suppl 1): 278–283.

19. Swift, A. (2015). One up, one over regional approach in "upper face: anatomy and regional approaches to injectables" found in the November 2015 supplement issue soft tissue fillers and neuromodulators: international and multidisciplinary perspectives. *Plast. Reconstr. Surg.* 136: 204S–218S.

20. Philipp-Dormston, W.G., Bieler, L., Hessenberger, M. et al. (2018). Intracranial penetration during temporal soft tissue filler injection – is it possible? *Dermatol. Surg.* 44: 84–91.

21. Sykes, J.M. (2009). Applied anatomy of the temporal region and forehead for injectable fillers. *J. Drugs Dermatol.* 8 (10 Suppl): s24–s27.

22. Tan, K.S., Oh, S.R., Priel, A. et al. (2011). Surgical anatomy of the forehead, eyelids, and midface for the aesthetic surgeon. In: *Master Techniques in Blepharoplasty and Periorbital Rejuvenation* (ed. G.G. Massry, M.R. Murphy and B. Azizzadeh), 11–24. Springer.

23. Hu, X.Z., Hu, J.Y., Wu, P.S. et al. (2016). Posterior ciliary artery occlusion caused by hyaluronic acid injections into the forehead: A case report. *Medicine* 95 (11): 1–4.

CHAPTER 4

The Eyebrow Revisited

B. Kent Remington[1] and Arthur Swift[2]
[1]Remington Laser Dermatology Centre, Calgary, Canada
[2]The Westmount Institute of Plastic Surgery, Montreal, QC, Canada

4.1 Introduction

The beautiful upper face is dependent on an attractive periorbital complex that includes youthful eyelids and an aesthetically appealing eyebrow. Many articles have been written about the aesthetics of the eyebrow with respect to facial shape, race, ethnicity, and cultural preferences [1–5]. The ideal eyebrow is challenging and complex to define because it is highly dynamic feature with changing shapes and positions that convey a myriad of expressions and emotions. The eyebrow is a floating structure whose position is determined by the opposing action of the frontalis muscle (elevator), and its antagonistic depressor muscles (procerus, corrugator supercilii, depressor supercilii, and orbicularis oculi) (Figure 4.1). Initially and exclusively the domain of the surgical brow lift, the introduction of cosmetic botulinum neurotoxin (BoNT) in the 1990s opened the door for non-surgical modalities to play a significant role in facial enhancement. In 2003, the authors presented the concept of individualizing the dose and location of BoNT into these mimetic muscles while underpinning the brow with filler to boost results beyond simple static elevation to definitive dynamic brow shaping, by moderating rather than obliterating movement [6]. With the amalgamation of volume restoring fillers, the aesthetic physician's palate of artistic therapies for eyebrow contouring has significantly expanded, establishing the procedure as a key element in beauty maximization.

The presence of unique eyebrow features such as length, height, and location of peak, or contrarily the total absence of the eyebrow, has a

Injectable Fillers: Facial Shaping and Contouring, Second Edition.
Edited by Derek H. Jones and Arthur Swift.
© 2019 John Wiley & Sons Ltd. Published 2019 by John Wiley & Sons Ltd.
Companion website: www.wiley.com/go/jones/injectable_fillers

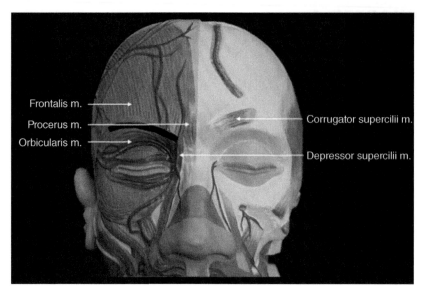

Frontalis m.
Procerus m.
Orbicularis m.
Corrugator supercilii m.
Depressor supercilii m.

Figure 4.1 Muscles affecting eyebrow position.

profound impact on attractiveness and perceived character. Infamous for her lack of eyebrow and eyelash hair, da Vinci's *Mona Lisa* is the best known and most written about painting in the world. Second only to her enigmatic smile, her lack of eyebrows has perplexed art aficionados for centuries. Never finished and unsigned, it is believed that da Vinci kept the *Mona Lisa* with him, continually working on it until his death a decade later, confirming his belief that 'art is never finished, only abandoned'. Mirroring da Vinci's philosophy of excellence, it must be affirmed that to raise a sagging eyebrow is virtuous; to contour it, divine.

4.2 Eyebrow Ageing

The periorbital complex typically shows signs of ageing in the mid-30s with skin colour and consistency changes (Figure 4.2). A quantitative analysis of periorbital ageing with 3-D surface imaging reveals a paradoxical finding that total eyebrow volume remains constant with age but there is a change in the relative ratio of fat to muscle content [7]. There is a decrease in the soft tissue/muscle volume but an increase in the fat content as revealed in 3-D reconstruction analysis using computed tomography (CT) scans of the face. In the younger individual, the major component of eyebrow volume is soft tissue and muscle, with only 18% of the volume consisting of fat. In the more mature patient, there is a significant increase in the galeal fat pad

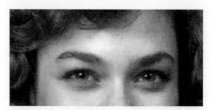

Figure 4.2 Early signs of periorbital ageing in a young female.

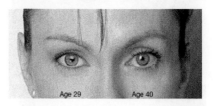

Figure 4.3 Split face photograph demonstrating upper eyelid arc change (see text) from age 29 to age 40 in a Caucasian female.

(including the retro-orbicularis oculi fat (ROOF)), which now represents 81% of brow volume [8].

There is a predictable resorption of facial bone with ageing that includes expansion of the superomedial and inferolateral aspects of the orbital rim [9]. This increase in orbital volume coupled with a relative decrease in intraorbital fat leads to a shift in the peak of the upper lid from medial to lateral, and the formation of an A-frame or infrabrow hollow in Caucasians (Figure 4.3), and a pan-upper eyelid volume loss in people of colour (Figure 4.4). Associated ageing skin changes and actinic damage (lines, creases, dyschromias, atrophy), volume loss at the soft tissue/muscle layer and bony remodelling create the appearance of progressive deflation of the entire region (Figure 4.5). The eyebrow loses its fullness, appears flattened, and lacks contour, making the supraorbital rim appear more prominent. The frontal bone is progressively remodelling with age, showing increased curvature of the upper forehead with flattening of the lower forehead and glabella in the mature individual (Figure 4.6). The loss of structure and support is evidenced by deflation of the head of the eyebrow, which contributes to dermatochalasia of the infrabrow medial canthal region.

Ageing therefore results in a change in location and contour of the eyebrow. Whereas gradual descent of the eyebrow with attendant dermatochalsia has been thought to be the exclusive pattern, it has become apparent that eyebrows can actually go up with age due to the interplay of frontalis muscle static dominance and bony orbital expansion (Figure 4.7). The deteriorated tissue of the region is more susceptible to the vectors of pull of the underlying muscles (dynamic discord), resulting in the variable positions of the entire eyebrow as seen in the elderly.

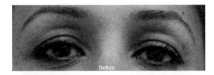

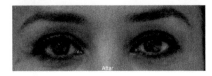

Figure 4.4 Upper eyelid (infrabrow) hollowing in a Persian female before and after correction with hyaluronic acid injection.

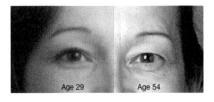

Figure 4.5 Split-face photograph demonstrating periorbital deflation with age (see text).

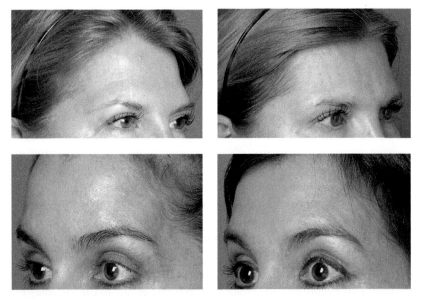

Figure 4.6 Increased convexity of the upper forehead and flattening of the lower forehead before and after treatment with hyaluronic acid.

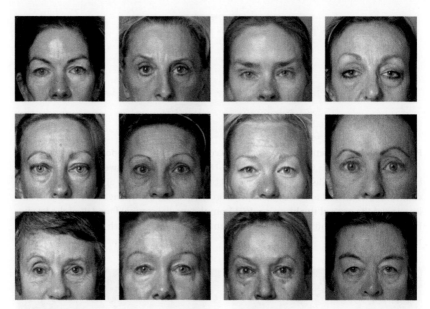

Figure 4.7 Mature females demonstrating naturally elevated eyebrow position.

4.3 Eyebrow Aesthetics

Eyebrow position and symmetry are an integral component of a youthful periorbital region, which remains one of the most important features defining facial beauty. Although varying in shape, thickness, and location from culture to culture and across periods in history, several gender-specific tenets grounded in mathematics endure regarding the aesthetic brow.

It must be appreciated that the eyebrow is a crucial component of the overall forehead/temple aesthetic unit, which should not be ignored in brow rejuvenation. The beautiful female forehead has a gentle convex ogee curve from trichon to supraorbital ridge which measures 12–14° from vertical, and the height of which measures Phi of the intercanthal distance (ICD) in the ideally proportioned face (Figure 4.8). A flattened or sloping brow greater than 15° from vertical is often undesirable for the female forehead, but acceptable in males. Although a detailed description is beyond the scope of this chapter, a pleasing convex appearance to the forehead can be easily fashioned by the subgaleal placement of volumizing filler (Figure 4.6).

From its origin overlying the supraorbital ridge, phi (0.618) of the ICD vertically above the medial canthus, the beautiful female eyebrow slopes upward and laterally at an angle of 10–20°, lying phi height from the pupil *above* the bony rim. Male brows are classically flatter, extending laterally *along* the supraorbital rim at 0–5° (Figure 4.9). Ideal eyebrow length in both genders should not exceed phi (1.618)

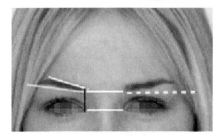

Figure 4.8 The aesthetic female eyebrow according to Golden proportions. (White = 1.0×; Black = 0.618×; Yellow = 1.618×). The distance between medial brows = intercanthal distance (ICD); medial brow begins vertically above medial canthus at height of 0.618 ICD; upslope of brow is 10–20; brow length is 1.618 ICD; location of the peak of the brow is = ICD from the medial canthal line; tail of the brow higher than medial end; fullness along the entire brow length which is essential under the lateral brow.

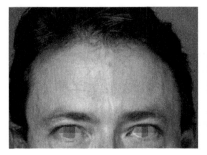 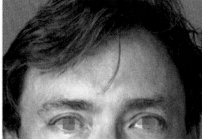

Figure 4.9 Male brow aesthetics before and after hyaluronic acid treatment for brow shaping and position.

of the ICD, which intersects a line drawn from the ipsilateral alar base obliquely through the lateral canthus.

The peak of the female brow is ideally located at the golden section of the brow length (0.618) which equals the ICD. This peak can also be determined by the point crossed by a line drawn from the alar base tangential to the lateral aspect of the pupil in the female. The male eyebrow typically is not as arched and has a less pronounced peak located more laterally at a point crossed by a line drawn from the alar base tangential to the lateral aspect of the iris. The female tail of the eyebrow should be situated at a height equal to or modestly higher than the medial segment, whereas the male eyebrow termination is more variable in height. Visualizing the tail of the brow on the anteroposterior (AP) view is aesthetically desirable and highly appreciated by patients when viewing themselves in the mirror. Excessive concavity of the temporal fossae is pathognomonic of advancing age, and can be restored to a slight concavity or a flat appearance in the female, thus preventing the tail of the eyebrow from 'disappearing around the corner'. Temple and forehead contouring are covered in excellent

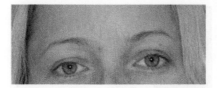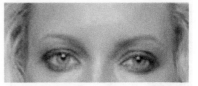

Figure 4.10 Creating an aesthetic female eyebrow to Golden proportions by the combination use of botulinum toxin and hyaluronic acid filler.

detail in Chapter 3 in this book; however, the authors' preferred technique as it relates to eyebrow shaping will be discussed in the following section on eyebrow treatment revisited.

A beautiful periorbital region demonstrates fullness of the entire eyebrow and infrabrow region in both genders. This is especially vital over the lateral supraorbital rim in the female to obscure the sharp bony features inferring masculinity. Cutaneous phi landmarks of the female aesthetic eyebrow are easily recognized and achievable in the clinical setting (Figure 4.10). Whereas a prominent supraorbital ridge is desirable in most males, excessive fullness of this promontory conveys masculinity in the female face.

The youthful infrabrow region exhibits upper lid fullness that follows the natural arc of the upper lid margin. For decades, classic blepharoplasty procedures consisted of aggressive removal of prominent intraorbital fat pads combined with redundant upper lid skin excision. This often resulted in a noticeable 'changed look' of excessive upper lid show when compared to the patient's younger morphology, or a hollow 'operated' appearance [10]. It has now become apparent that volume replenishment of the ageing infrabrow is a crucial component of periorbital rejuvenation, either as a standalone procedure or coupled with surgery.

4.4 Eyebrow Treatment Revisited

Fullness of the supraorbital brow and upper lid can be achieved by the modest use of hyaluronic acid (HA) filler using needle or cannula technique. Hyaluronic acids are the authors' products of choice because of the reliability, consistency and reversibility of results. The goal is even fill distribution over the entire length of the brow that obscures the supraorbital rim and creates a contour that flows in a gentle arc medially to the radix of the nose. Injection of HA at the supraorbital crest will force the eyebrow up if the brow is above the promontory. The opposite holds true for injections of HA at the supraorbital crest that will force the eyebrow down when the latter is below

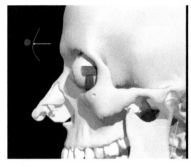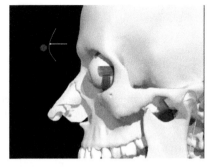

Figure 4.11 Injections on the supraorbital rim can displace the brow up or down depending on its position relative to the promontory. (see text).

the promontory (Figure 4.11). This effect is similar to that seen on the nipple-areolar complex (NAC) during breast enhancement surgery depending on the location of the maximal projection of the implant relative to the NAC.

The authors describe a five step filler approach to eyebrow restoration that is preceded by neuromodulator brow shaping (Figure 4.12).

1. High G′ product under the head of the brow on periosteum to lift and contour.
2. Intermediate G′ product with cannula under the body of the eyebrow.
3. Low G′ product with cannula for infrabrow hollowing or A-frame deformity.
4. High G′ product for the tail of the brow on the superolateral orbital rim periosteum.
5. High or intermediate G′ product for temporal hollowing and lateral tail of brow position.

1. *Head of the Brow*
   Placement of higher G′ sub-brow filler in this region is of high risk due to the presence of the supratrochlear artery, commonly located under the most medial crease of the corrugator supercilii (see Chapter 1). Product must be deposited *on the periosteum* away from the crease, preferably by blunt lateral cannula technique, although fine needle injections are possible in experienced hands, where aspiration and slow injection are mandatory. Quantities in the order of $0.1 \, cm^3$ suffice, followed by gentle moulding to create a flowing arc towards the radix of the nose (Figure 4.13).
2. *Body of the Eyebrow*
   Use of intermediate G′ HA is recommended from a lateral approach on periosteum with a blunt-tipped cannula of 27G or thicker. The preferred port of entry of the cannula should be overlying the lateral supraorbital rim and the product deposited in an antegrade fashion.

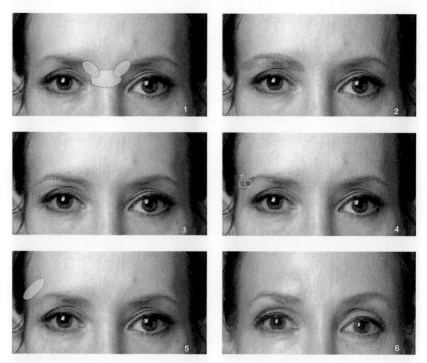

Figure 4.12 5Five-step approach to filler contouring of the eyebrow (1–5; see text). Final result (6).

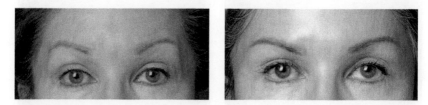

Figure 4.13 Treatment of a deflated head of the brow with hyaluronic acid filler creating a natural arc to the nasal radix.

This insertion point can then be used for access to the infrabrow hollow with a thinner product, limiting the possibility of globe injury due to the cantilever effect of the underlying bone. With the thumb and index of the free hand isolating the eyebrow, $0.2\,cm^3$ of intermediate HA is typically required to achieve a pleasing contour (Figure 4.14). Slightly more product in the predetermined region of the eyebrow apex, followed by gentle moulding with cool ultrasound gel, can create an aesthetically pleasing result.

3. *Infrabrow Hollow*

As previously mentioned, the authors' experience has revealed that hollowing of the infrabrow region can appear as an A-frame deformity,

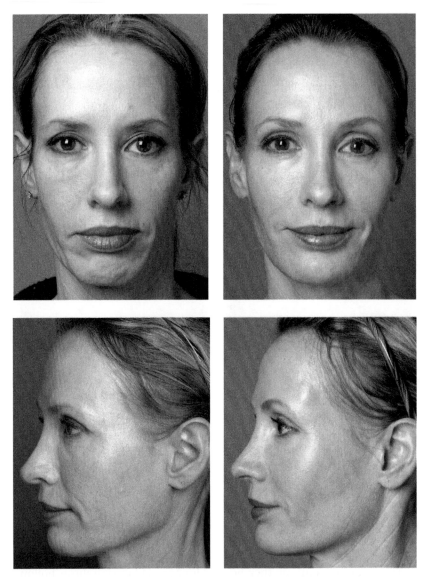

Figure 4.14 Filler along the length to the body of the eyebrow as part of the comprehensive approach to full face 'BeautiPHIcation'.

commonly seen in Caucasians, or as a complete crescenteric hollowing above the upper eyelid, as seen more commonly in Asians, in people of colour, and in people of Mediterranean descent. Injections of the infrabrow should create upper lid fullness that follows the natural arc of the upper lid margin (Figure 4.15).

Infrabrow hollows are best treated with a thin low G′ HA that is easily spread and moulded below the supraorbital ridge. A cannula is

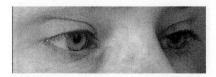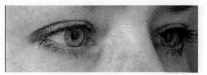

Figure 4.15 Treatment of the infrabrow with hyaluronic acid, creating a natural fold that follows the ciliary margin of the upper lid.

selected of appropriate length to reach the medial canthal region, and of significant gauge (27G or thicker) to minimize the risk of penetration of vital structures of the region (e.g. vessels, globe). Employing a port of entry over the superolateral orbital rim and cantilevering the cannula off of the bone, can prevent inadvertent retroseptal penetration. This is critical as inadvertent deposition of HA behind the orbital septum has been implicated in repeated and persistent periorbital oedema. The cannula must advance with little resistance and minimal pain, gliding in the subdermal plane of the infrabrow region immediately inferior to the supraorbital bone (Figure 4.11). The index of the free hand is used to palpate and monitor the position of the tip of the instrument while gently moulding the deposition of product. Slow antegrade and retro-grade injection of minute quantities of HA (totalling less than 0.25 cm³) can re-create a youthful fold following the arc of the upper eyelashes. During treatment, the syringe is uncoupled from the cannula, which is left *in situ*, and the patient is placed in an upright sitting position to assess the aesthetic result and need for any further refinements.

The authors prefer to use low G′ HA that has been previously 'wetted down' with lidocaine or saline in a 1 : 1 blend in the perior-bital zone, thereby priming the HA with the hydration it seeks, and consequently limiting post-treatment swelling.

4. *Tail of the Eyebrow (Vertical Lift)*
    The position and visibility of the tail of the brow is vital to the overall aesthetic of the region. Deposition of higher G′ HA onto the supraorbital rim by needle or cannula can create the desirable Fabergé egg fullness of the region and *vertically elevate* a depressed tail creating a sharper peak to the eyebrow (Figure 4.16). Typically, 0.1–0.2 cm³ is adequate to achieve this effect. Fullness in this area may exacerbate previously existing hol-lowing of the adjacent temple, the treatment of which must always be considered when augmenting the volume of the bony lateral orbit.

5. *Tail of Eyebrow (Lateral Lift) and Temple*
    If a tail of brow that is elevated and splayed laterally is the desired aesthetic, then addition of volume to a hollowed temple is the procedure of choice (Figure 4.17). Safe correction of overly scaph-oid temporal hollows with simultaneous positioning of the tail of the

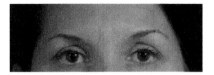 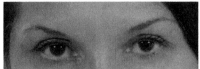

Figure 4.16 Treatment of the A-frame deformity by infrabrow injections of hyaluronic acid. Simultaneous injections of filler onto the lateral promontory resulted in elevation of the tail of the brow (see text).

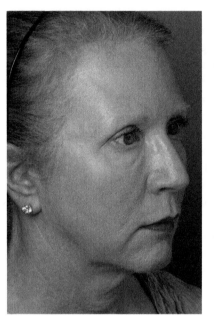 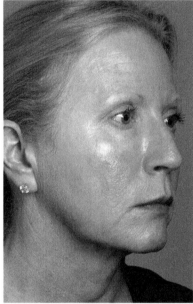

Figure 4.17 Treatment of temple hollowing with filler resulting in a lateral elevation of the both the tail of the brow and the sub-brow hooding.

eyebrow can be achieved only through a solid understanding of the injection anatomy of the region. For the purposes of tail of eyebrow positioning, planned temporal injection is a single puncture vertically oriented *down to bone*, 1 cm up the temporal fusion line and 1 cm lateral, parallel to the supraorbital rim (one up, one over), as described in Chapter 1. A hyaluronic acid (HA) of high or intermediate G' and cohesive character is selected, with the goal to 'reflate' the *aesthetic* temporal hollow by creating a tent pole and overlying canopy with one single injection.

Typically, 0.3–0.6 cm³ is required to achieve a pleasing contour while simultaneously repositioning the tail of the eyebrow. The reader is referred to Chapter 1 on facial anatomy for an in-depth discussion of the authors' preferred procedure. Patient satisfaction is noted to be high, as rather than disappearing around the corner and falling into the hollow of the temple, the beautiful aspect of the tail of the brow is now visible when looking in the mirror on the AP view.

The aesthetic goal of temple fill in the female is to maintain a flat or slightly concave/convex curvature to the temple region. Excessive convexity signifies large muscle mass and is a masculinizing feature which must be avoided.

4.5 Summary

If the eyes are commonly referred to as the windows of the soul, then the eyebrow is the frame of humanity, emotion, personality, and empathy. With prolonged habit plus genetics, the frowning negative expressions of the stress of life can become present even at rest, but are more obvious with animation, giving an angry – worried – upset – annoyed – stressed appearance that often has little to do with the actual demeanour of the patient. For over 25 years, neuromodulators have been used to obliterate glabellar lines in an attempt to soften the patient's severe look. In the early years of neuromodulators, most aesthetic injectors did not taken advantage of the anatomical studies of the glabellar complex and the variable contribution of these muscles to the position of the medial head of the brow – the aim was to eliminate the frown zones with no attention to what the eyebrows were doing or what they looked like after treatment. The 'Spock brow' became the new norm. In the late 1990s, injection specialists began elevating the eyebrows with neuromodulators to create what was called the 'Botox® Brow Lift' by relaxing the eyebrow depressors so the static contribution of the frontalis muscle to eyebrow position was dominant. Starting in 2003, the authors began 'shaping' the eyebrows with precise injections of BoNT and then adding HA fillers to underpin and help shape the brows, incorporating cannulas in 2010 and by design – by choice – re-creating the peak of the feminine eyebrow predetermined by the Golden Mean phi callipers.

With ageing, exposure to both ultraviolet and infrared radiation, habitual smoking, and contact with pollution result in the facial skin deteriorating at a faster rate than the diminishing strength of the underlying mimetic muscles. The repetitive movements of blinking, squinting, and facial expressions further compound the facial envelope's waning structure, leading to both a static and dynamic discord of eyebrow position and movement. As for other areas of the face, the artistic use of filler and neuromodulator can restore the proportion, harmony, and balance of youth to the eyebrow region.

Feminizing the eyebrow in the female patient is one of the more rewarding restoration projects, both for the syringe therapist and the patient. This
is usually a serendipitous experience for patients as they are often unaware
of the gradual negative changes in eyebrow position and shape. Even
in those faces that have won the genetic DNA lottery, eyebrow shaping
further enhances facial harmony, balance, and proportion. No longer the
focus of isolated toxin therapy, non-surgical eyebrow shaping can best be
accomplished by the synergy of neuromodulator and filler (Figure 4.18).

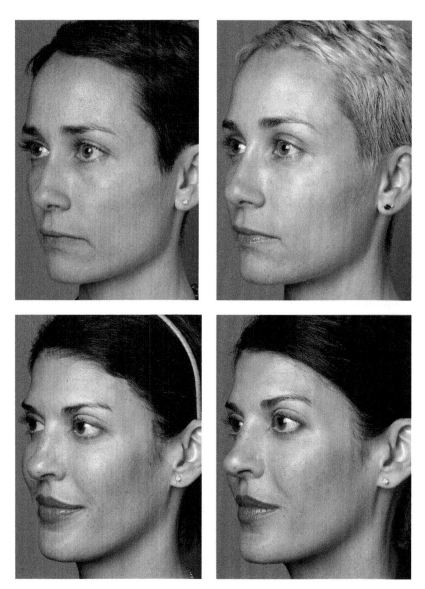

Figure 4.18 Eyebrow shaping and positioning as part of the comprehensive approach
to facial 'BeautiPHIcation'.

References

1. Delyzer, T.L. and Yazdani, A. (2013 Fall). Characterizing the lateral slope of the aging female eyebrow. *The Canadian Journal of Plastic Surgery* 21 (3): 173–177.
2. Schreiber, J.E., Singh, N.K., and Klatsky, S.A. (2005 Jul–Aug). Beauty lies in the "eyebrow" of the beholder: a public survey of eyebrow aesthetics. *Aesthetic Surgery Journal* 25 (4): 348–352.
3. Yalcinkaya, E., Cingi, C., Soken, H. et al. (2016 Feb). Aesthetic analysis of the ideal eyebrow shape and position. *European Archives of Oto-Rhino-Laryngology* 273 (2): 305–310.
4. Baker, S.B., Dayan, J.H., Crane, A., and Kim, S. (2007 Jun). The influence of brow shape on the perception of facial form and brow aesthetics. *Plastic and Reconstructive Surgery* 119 (7): 2240–2247.
5. Alex, J.C. (2004 Aug). Aesthetic considerations in the elevations of the eyebrow. *Facial Plastic Surgery* 20 (3): 193–198.
6. Remington, K.; Swift, A., Brow shaping with botulinum toxin. Presented at the Allergan F.A.C.E. Symposium, Las Vegas, 2003.
7. Camp, M.C., Wong, W.W., Filip, Z. et al. (2011). A quantitative analysis of periorbital aging with three-dimensional surface imaging. *Journal of Plastic, Reconstructive & Aesthetic Surgery* 64: 148–154.
8. Papageorgiou, K.I., Mancini, R., Garneau, H.C. et al. (2012). Paradoxical finding: female eyebrow fat pad volume increases with age. *Aesthetic Surgery Journal* 32 (1): 46–57.
9. Shaw, R.B. Jr. and Kahn, D.M. (2007). Aging of the midface bony elements: a three-dimensional computed tomographic study. *Plastic and Reconstructive Surgery* 119: 675.
10. Ciuci, P. and Obagi, S. (2008 Aug). Rejuvenation of the periorbital complex with autologous fat transfer. *Journal of Oral and Maxillofacial Surgery* 6 (8): 1686–1693.

CHAPTER 5

Periorbital Rejuvenation

Arthur Swift[1] and Herve Raspaldo[2]
[1]The Westmount Institute of Plastic Surgery, Montreal, QC, Canada
[2]Private Practice Facial Surgeon, Geneva, Switzerland

5.1 The Aesthetic Periorbital Complex

The periorbital complex (POC) consists of the eyebrow and supraorbital rim, the infrabrow and upper eyelid, the lateral canthus, the lower eyelid, and the infraorbital rim/upper cheek junction (Figure 5.1). Regardless of race or ethnicity, beauty of the region (Figure 5.2) relies on an upper periorbital volume that is essential in creating fullness of the infrabrow region and upper lid sulcus. There should be even fat distribution over the entire length of the brow that obscures the supraorbital rim and the upper lid fullness should follow the natural arc of the upper lid ciliary margin. The aesthetic eyebrow is covered in greater detail in Chapter 4 in this text.

The ideal lower periorbital contour displays a mild lower lid convexity, short vertical height, and fullness obscuring the infraorbital rim. A youthful lateral canthal region has a smooth contour that is slightly concave with no bony rim show and lies 5–10° higher than the medial canthus, creating a slight upward slant to the palpebral fissure. There should be zero to minimal scleral show below the iris, and a smooth eyelid cheek continuum. The harmonious infraorbital region therefore exhibits a single convexity of youth (positive vector) with the skin taught and smooth without redundancy.

Tear troughs can be evident during childhood as a genetic display of infraorbital anatomy and are therefore not truly defects (Figure 5.3). The commonly referred to 'tear trough deformity' is actually a *revealing of anatomy* with senescent loss of fat that occurs with maturity as early as

Injectable Fillers: Facial Shaping and Contouring, Second Edition.
Edited by Derek H. Jones and Arthur Swift.
© 2019 John Wiley & Sons Ltd. Published 2019 by John Wiley & Sons Ltd.
Companion website: www.wiley.com/go/jones/injectable_fillers

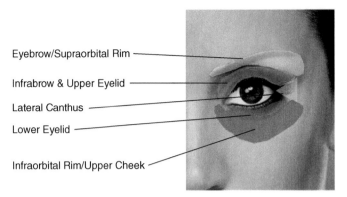

Eyebrow/Supraorbital Rim

Infrabrow & Upper Eyelid

Lateral Canthus

Lower Eyelid

Infraorbital Rim/Upper Cheek

Figure 5.1 The aesthetic components of the periorbital complex.

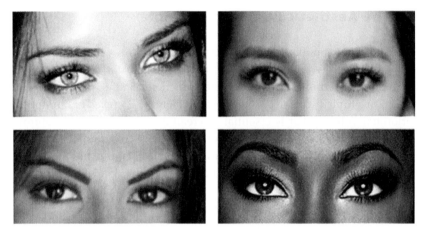

Figure 5.2 The universally beautiful periorbital complex.

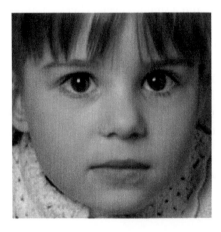

Figure 5.3 The appearance of congenital 'tear troughs' in childhood. Source: Photo courtesy of Dr. K. Remington.

the third decade of life. It is characterized by tone and texture changes in the infraorbital region and a sunken, sullen appearance that makes the individual look tired and aged.

Eyelids not only serve a crucial reflexive function in protecting the globe from foreign material as well as assisting in visual accommodation and sheltering the retina from excessively bright light, but also contribute immeasurably to overall facial beauty. Our natural tendency when greeting individuals is initially to engage eye contact (perhaps an evolutionary response to assessing friend or foe) from which our gaze then spreads peripherally [1]. Volume replacement with filler or autologous fat in the periorbital complex is highly challenging due to the delicate nature of the area. Any small irregularity or lump underlying the thin skin of the region is not only immediately visible but may actually interfere with the subtle dynamic of eye expression (blinking, smiling, etc.). Certainly, a very detailed understanding of the underlying anatomy is essential to avoid inadvertent intravascular injections that can lead to blindness.

This chapter introduces an algorithm for systematic assessment and subsequent injection of hyaluronic acid (HA) fillers for the treatment of periorbital hollowing based on a novel segmentation of tear trough anatomy, 'safer' injection planes, and the quality (tone and texture) of overlying skin. This approach was developed from a better understanding of the physiology of the ageing process and volume loss, a more detailed clinical evaluation of existing signs of ageing, and an appreciation of individual anatomical variations and the contribution of periorbital rejuvenation to overall midface beauty.

5.2 Periorbital Anatomy

The three-dimensional aspect of the face can be considered as heart-shaped as it relates to functional anatomy and volume. Each layer of the face has its specific influence on facial morphology. Consequently, it is essential for the injection specialist to determine which anatomical component is responsible for facial disharmony prior to selecting the appropriate technique for its correction.

The facial muscles surrounded by deep fat and overlying subcutaneous soft tissue cover an irregular facial skeleton that is very different in each patient. Anatomical variations are seen in fat content, bone thickness, the coursing of nerves and vessels, and the prominence of salivary glands. Varying thickness of fat must harmoniously fill the face to provide for a youthful appearance.

The muscles of facial expression have a common embryologic origin from the second branchial/pharyngeal arch, are innervated by the VIIth nerve, and are organized into superficial and deep layers. They include the occipitofrontalis, temporoparietalis, procerus, nasalis (transverse and dilator nares portions), depressor septi nasi, orbicularis oculi, corrugator supercilii, depressor supercilii, auricular triad (anterior, posterior, and superior), orbicularis oris, depressor anguli oris, risorius, zygomaticus major and minor, levator labii superioris, levator anguli oris, levator labii superioris alaeque nasi, depressor labii inferioris, buccinator (aids in smiling), and mentalis (Figure 5.4). The superficial muscles of facial expression are very thin (1–2 mm), long and flat, and are located immediately below the overlying skin to which they adhere (e.g. orbicularis oculi). Deeper below this superficial layer lie the shorter and stronger mimetic muscles which, in combination with their superficial counterparts, are responsible for expressing 21 emotional states [2].

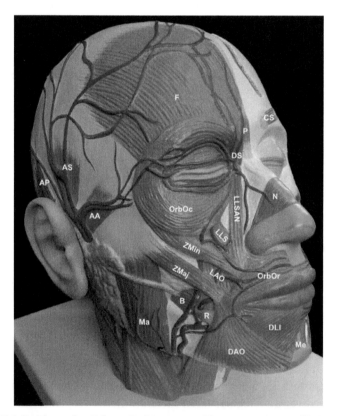

Figure 5.4 Facial muscles: F, frontalis; P, procerus; CS, corrugator supercilii; DS, depressor supercilii; OrbOc, orbicularis oculi; LLSAN, levator labii superioris alequae nasii; N, nasalis; AP, auricularis posterioris; AS, auricularis superioris; AA, auricularis anterioris; ZMin, zygomaticus minor; ZMaj, zygomatic major; LLS, levator labii superioris; LAO, levator anguli oris; B, buccinator; R, risorius [sectioned]; Ma, masseter; DAO, depressor anguli oris; DLI, depressor labii inferioris; Me, mentalis; OrbOr, orbicularis oris.

The *orbicularis oculi muscle* is the only muscle capable of closing the eye and consists of the palperbral (pretarsal and preseptal) and orbital portions. A lacrimal section that facilitates the pumping of tears into the lacrimal sac has been described, which may represent extensions of the pretarsal and preseptal orbicularis. The muscle is firmly adherent to the periosteum medially at its tear trough origin from medial canthus to medial iris, as well as at its insertion laterally into the periosteum at the palpebral raphe. The tear trough ligament is a true oseocutaneous ligament consistently found between the palpebral and orbital portions of the orbicularis muscle and contributes to the prominence of the 'deformity' that bears its name [3, 4]. More laterally, the orbicularis retaining ligament (orbitomalar ligament) is another true retaining ligament of the face as it originates from the periosteum of the orbital rim and traverses the orbicularis muscle to insert into the skin of the lid–cheek junction. However, most of the non-adherent, aviator-glasses-shaped orbicularis glides over the medial and lateral suborbicularis oculi fat pad (SOOF), allowing for a sphincteric action with eyelid closure (Figure 5.5). It is in this deep fat plane (SOOF) where precise amounts of HA (or fat) can recreate a young periorbital and subpalpebral contour [5]. It is also with the understanding that the *medial* orbicularis is firmly adherent to the underlying infraorbital bony rim that injection of filler on bone in this region results in intramuscular deposition, as will be further described later in this chapter.

The eyelids have no subcutaneous fat, whereas the malar fat pad is composed of a thick layer of subcutaneous fat extending from the malar eminence to the nasolabial crease.

(a)   (b)

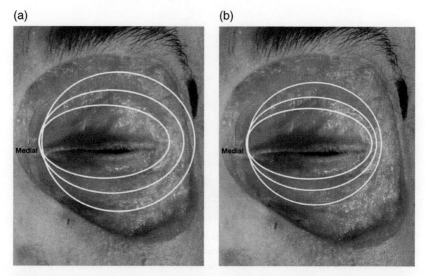

Figure 5.5 The aviator-glasses-shaped orbicularis oculi showing the medial zones of bony adherence (grey). Schematic at rest (a) and during sphincteric contraction (b).

The vascular anatomy surrounding the orbit is a minefield of arteries and veins representing the confluence between the internal and external carotid systems. Terminal cutaneous branches of the ophthalmic artery include the supraorbital artery (SOA), supratrochlear artery (STA), the dorsal nasal artery, and the zygomatic artery branches of the lacrimal artery. These arteries have numerous anastomoses with the external carotid system: the superficial temporal with the SOA and/or the STA; the transverse facial artery and deep temporal arteries with the zygomatic branches of the lacrimal artery; the inferior orbital artery and the angular artery with the dorsal nasal artery. The injection specialist must take note that the infraorbital foramen and its neurovascular bundle is located 5–10 mm below the infraorbital bony rim at approximately the vertical level of the medial iris (80%) or more laterally as far as the mid-pupil (20%) [6]. The foramen is angled inferiorly providing a hood of bone superiorly which protects these vital structures from a lateral approaching cannula, but because of the inverted funnel shape of the medial maxilla, the foramen is inviting from an inferior approach (Figure 5.6). The venous system surrounding the orbit is no less complex and variable.

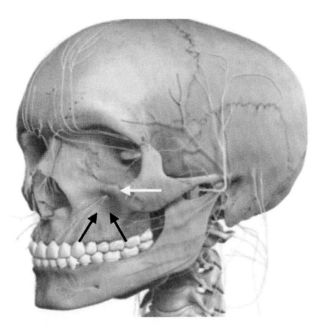

Figure 5.6 The body of the maxilla is shaped like an inverted funnel with its apex at the infraorbital foramen. An inferior approach with cannula or needle can easily enter the foramen (black arrows). The neurovascular bundle and foramen are angled inferiorly, making a lateral approach with cannula (white arrow) the safer technique for medial subpalpebral filler.

Treatment of midface ageing is covered elsewhere in this text. However, it must be emphasized that when treating the midface area, the injector must take into consideration the facial artery entering the face from under the mandible just medial to the masseter's anterior border (Figure 5.4). This major artery then runs deeply on the buccinator muscle under the muscles of facial expression towards the pyriform region of the maxilla at the top of the nasolabial fold. Its common communication with the angular artery results in a direct access to the internal carotid system branches around the orbital rim as outlined earlier.

5.3 Pathophysiology of Periorbital Ageing

Nomenclature regarding the infraorbital region is confusing when describing the clinical presentations of periorbital ageing. The authors prefer to use the term tear trough to refer to the hollow groove extending from the medial canthus to the medial iris (ending just below the infraorbital rim) (Figure 5.7). The term infraorbital crescent or hollow refers to the C-shaped depression present along the entire infraorbital rim. The term nasojugal groove for the purpose of this chapter is reserved for the lid–cheek junction that extends below the orbital rim and overlies the orbitomalar ligament. The term infrabrow hollowing refers to the A-frame deformity of the upper orbit typical in the ageing Caucasian (Figure 5.28b), as well as the pan-upper eyelid volume depletion typically seen in the ageing Asian and Persian face (Figure 5.29a).

One of the cardinal signs of ageing is the outward appearance of tissue sagging [7], both apparent and true. Observations on periorbital and midface ageing have shown there to be very little ptosis (inferior descent) of the *lid–cheek junction* or of the *upper* midface. The phenomenon of apparent descent is probably due to the contrast of tone and texture changes in

(a)   (b)   (c)

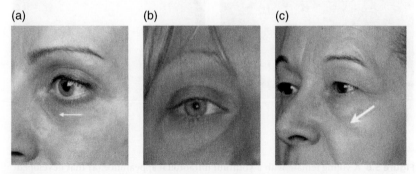

Figure 5.7 (a) Tear trough; (b) infraorbital hollow or crescent; (c) nasojugal groove (see text).

the skin [8]. The remaining facial envelope descends from changes in all anatomical layers including bone resorption and remodelling, loss of dermal collagen and elastin, stretching of ligamentous structures, thinning of muscles, and loss of fat compartment volume, regardless of compounding environmental factors [9].

Ageing of the tear trough results from a myriad of factors, including dynamic and volumetric changes. Beyond the toxic stress of ultraviolet radiation, air pollution, and smoking, the thin eyelid skin is subjected (approximately 1200 times per hour) to the repetitive accordion contraction of blinking/squinting. The volume of the tear trough is composed of the underlying musculature (origins of the levator muscles of the lip; the pretarsal and preseptal orbicularis oculi muscle), the superficial fat pad, and the deep (SOOF) fat compartment, all of which atrophy with age. This is further accentuated by the senescent tone and texture changes that occur in the overlying skin. Static and dynamic wrinkles are therefore intensified by the periorbital skin being overwhelmed by the contraction of the underlying orbicularis muscle.

The appearance of lower eyelid intraorbital fat herniation (Figure 5.8) heralds a tired appearance and is only partially related to an attenuated septum and orbicularis muscle. Opposing theories are well documented regarding the aetiology of these lower lid 'eyebags' as cause [10, 11] (fat herniation precedes globe descent) or effect [12, 13] (a stretched Lockwood's ligament causes globe descent forcing the fat forward).

As mentioned previously, the youthful inferior orbital region is a single slightly convex curve from lid to cheek. With ageing, a double convexity occurs and festooning of lower-eyelid skin may appear due to fluid retention over the malar prominence (Figure 5.9). Many aetiologies for malar oedema have been described, including waning lymphatic drainage and prolapse of

(a)   (b)

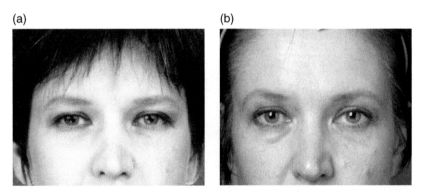

Figure 5.8 A young female with a youthful infraorbital appearance (a) that developed lower eyelid intraorbital fat herniation ('eye bags') with age (b). Source: Reproduced with permission from K. Remington.

(a)   (b)

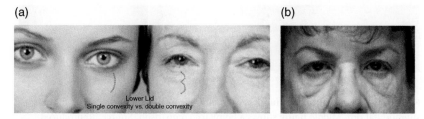

Figure 5.9 (a) Change in lower lid convexity with age; (b) infraorbital festoons (malar oedema).

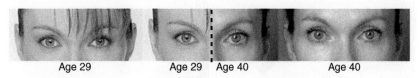

Age 29   Age 29   Age 40   Age 40

Figure 5.10 Upper eyelid arc change with age exhibiting peak movement from a medial to a central location. The middle figure shows a hemiface comparison. Source: Reproduced with permission from K. Remington.

the SOOF through rents or gaps in the orbicularis muscle causing inefficient muscle contribution to the pumping out of fluid in the region [14].

Ageing of the upper periorbital area may reflect depletion of the soft tissue as well as bony resorption of the orbit, giving rise to a sunken appearance [15]. A quantitative analysis of periorbital ageing with three-dimensional surface imaging has revealed a consistent loss of fat at the superomedial orbit, nasojugal groove, and palpebral-malar junction averaging $0.8\,cm^3$ over 28 years [16]. The upper eyelid arc changes, with the peak moving from a medial to central location (Figure 5.10). Loss or paucity of the subcutaneous fat often leads to a gaunt and unattractive appearance pathognomonic of the ageing orbit. Interestingly, three-dimensional reconstruction analysis using CT scans has shown that there is a paradoxical increase in female eyebrow fat pad volume with age [17]. There is no change in *total* eyebrow volume, as the decrease in soft tissue/ muscle volume is offset by an increase in fat volume (81% of the eyebrow volume in the elderly female consists of fat). The eyebrow therefore loses its *structural* fullness and appears deflated, contributing to supraorbital rim prominence and upper eyelid dermatochalasia (Figure 5.11).

Typically, facial ageing in the adult is marked by a horizontal increase in the size of the craniofacial skeleton in both men and women, including head circumference, length, and bizygomatic width [18]. This can occur in parallel with changes in anterior facial height [19–23]. Anterior–posterior (sagittal) changes are complex, but tend to be characterized by a decrease in craniofacial skeletal size, possibly related to alveolar bone changes [24]. Areas with a strong predisposition to remodel include the

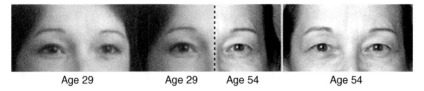

Age 29   Age 29   Age 54   Age 54

Figure 5.11 Loss of structural fullness of the infrabrow causing prominence of the supraorbital rim. Middle figure shows a hemiface comparison. Source: Reproduced with permission from K. Remington.

(a)   (b)

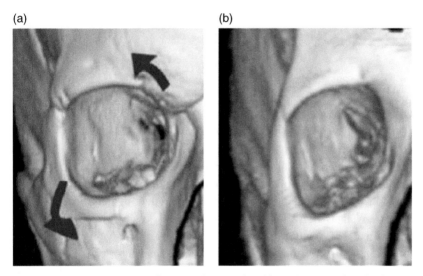

Figure 5.12 Orbital expansion from youth (a) to the elderly (b). IOF, infraorbital foramen.

midface skeleton, particularly the maxilla. The pyriform region of the nose recedes backwards and upwards, and the superomedial and infero-lateral aspects of the orbital rim 'expand' outwards (Figure 5.12) [25]. The increase in orbital aperture size with age in both sexes causes a relative senile enophthalmos with loss of the globe's curving effect on the lower lid (Figure 5.13). The enlarged orbit is often evidenced by a higher position of the eyebrow relative to the globe (Figures 5.13 and 5.14). The downward displacement of the lateral canthal tendon with bone remodelling also leads to a flattening of the youthful 5–10° canthal slant from medial to lateral (Figure 5.14). There are ethnic variations that should be noted, as a greater relative descent of the lateral canthal complex has been re-ported in African Americans [26]. Furthermore, the orbicularis muscle dominates the deteriorated periorbital skin ('dynamic discord') causing a squinting and decreased interlimbal show ('small eye') with smiling (Figure 5.14).

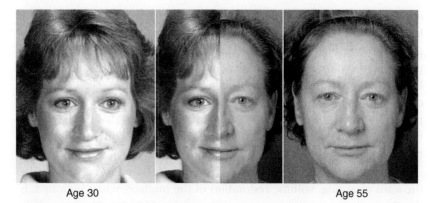

Age 30   Age 55

Figure 5.13 Senile enophthalmos with loss of the lower lid curvature. Source: Reproduced with permission from K. Remington.

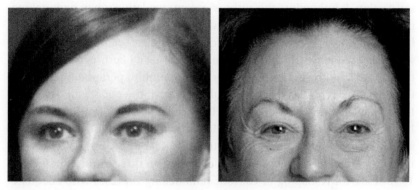

Figure 5.14 Eyebrow elevation and 'small eye' seen with age (see text). Source: Reproduced with permission from K. Remington.

5.4 Enhancing the Periorbital Region

The youthful face is typically considered the gold standard of cosmetic intervention, as evidenced by fullness of features, smooth contours, gradual transitions, highlighted features with appropriate hollows or shadows, and a full and wide midface. The aesthetic of the periorbital region, however, is much more complex in that it must radiate youth, beauty, and a rested look. As for all facial cosmetic interventions, restoring the ageing face should be in the context of what is age-appropriate – a 'best version of self'. Creating beauty creates youth, but the corollary may not hold true. The 'ideal' facial volume in a 25-year-old individual is not appropriate when 55 years old as the skeletal platform has remodelled with age. Thus, practitioners need to focus on proportion and contours while staying within the boundaries of what is aesthetically appropriate for the patient's age. Repeated or excessive volumizing may lead to unsightly swelling in an elderly patient whose marginal lymphatic flow is further taxed by the accumulation of fluid due to the presence of hygroscopic HA fillers. This is nowhere more evident than in the periorbital region, where the 'personality' of the selected filler is on display under the thin skin of the region. Aesthetic contouring of the periorbital region requires sublime technical prowess ('a light hand') as the area portends the highest rate of undesirable results, the majority of which are injector related.

Although the eyes are generally the first facial area to be affected by the signs of ageing, volume restoration of the midface, when indicated, is the first essential step in tear trough correction [27, 28]. The immediate rejuvenation effect and improved skin radiance not only has a significant positive impact on the facial aesthetic but also on patient motivation and satisfaction. It is therefore the authors' recommendation when undertaking periorbital rejuvenation to first assess and correct any concomitant midface volume loss (Figure 5.15). This can become part of a comprehensive, systematic sequence of full-face beautification using both neurotoxin and filler [29–31] proceeding from midface restoration to periorbital rejuvenation to perioral enhancement, and culminating in the remodelling of other features such as eyebrow, eye frame, forehead, nose, and lips (Figure 5.16). In selected cases, the typical volume loss that is pathognomonic of midface ageing may not be present, necessitating surgical or non-surgical interventions to address the patient's needs, depending on three distinct strategies:

1. A desire for reshaping or contour remodelling (in cases with adequate volume) by rhytidectomy and blepharoplasty techniques, or with energy devices in less severe cases.

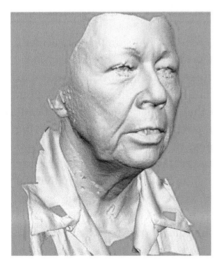

Figure 5.15 Correction of tear troughs alone producing a suboptimal aesthetic result in a patient with significant midface volume loss.

(a)   (b)

(c)   (d)

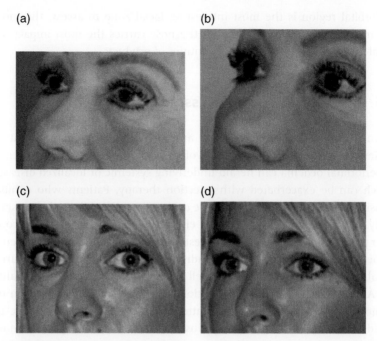

Figure 5.16 Simultaneous correction of midface and periorbital volume loss creating a rested, beautiful, youthful appearance.

(a)   (b)

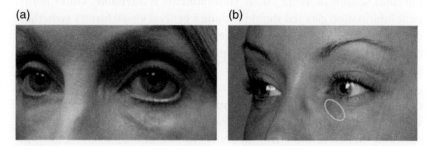

Figure 5.17 (a) Lower lid ectropion and injection nodules of the infraorbital region; (b) Tyndall effect of infraorbital HA filler.

2. A desire for refilling (in cases of soft tissue loss or inadequate volume) via autologous fat grafting or injectable dermal fillers [32, 33].

3. A desire for smoothing of wrinkled skin through ablative laser therapy, chemical peels, dermal fillers, or platelet-rich plasma injections.

As midface volumetric enhancement is covered elsewhere in this text, this chapter will focus on the authors' experience with injectable HA treatment of the periorbital region.

The periorbital area is the most difficult zone to correct with injectable fillers as sequelae of injection are often evident. Every filler has its own personality, which can be revealed under the stress of repetitive contractions behind the overlying thin skin (Figure 5.17). To the contrary, the periorbital region is the most interesting facial zone to assess, the most rewarding to treat, and along with the nose carries the most impact for facial beautification using small quantities of products.

5.5 Consultation and Assessment

At consultation, a thorough history and physical exam is paramount to achieving satisfactory results and avoiding adverse events. The presence of periorbital oedema can herald underlying systemic or localized disease, which can be exacerbated with injection therapy. Patients who exhibit transitory cyclical swelling during the day, unilateral or bilateral, are especially susceptible to the hygroscopic effects of HA. Clinicians should consider performing a thyroid function test prior to treatment in those patients suspected of thyroid-related eye conditions. A review of skin issues (urticarial, erythema, rosacea, etc.) as well as a medication history is warranted. Although not mandatory, cessation of blood thinning medication or homoeopathy for one week pretreatment is advisable when possible to avoid unsightly bruising. In those instances where anticoagulants must be maintained, prior icing of the region, immediate pressure post-injection, choice of cannulas or thin-gauge needles, and scheduling of the injection session to avoid public commitments is advisable. Other pertinent information gleaned should include a general visual history (whether corrective lenses are necessary for near or far vision), the presence of dry or teary eye syndrome, and the frequency of infections (blepharitis, conjunctivitis, herpes simplex).

The examination of the region must include a standard evaluation of the eyelids (e.g. presence of upper lid ptosis, scleral show, etc.) as well as a 'squinch test' to determine orbicularis function and a 'snap-back test' to determine lower lid laxity (to rule out senile ectropion). In patients with a history of previous injection therapy of known product, palpation can determine the presence or absence of retained filler that may react with the planned treatment. The authors consider a history of prior injections of indeterminate origin or 'permanent' filler in the region, which may be 'disturbed and activated', as a relative contraindication to injection therapy. Although some success has been possible in camouflaging previous inadequate treatment (Figure 5.31c and d), the instillation of a relatively benign blended HA can trigger inflammation in existing product. The injector should also take note of any previous blepharoplasty surgery (transconjunctival or subciliary) that may have altered the local anatomy (e.g. adhered vessels; released ligaments) and created a rigid scarred bed.

5.6 Injection Rationale

The injection techniques described below are personal and based on the authors' 20-plus years familiarity with dermal fillers as well as their substantial experience with periorbital plastic surgery.

As emphasized previously, treatment of the periocular region remains challenging due to noticeable swelling, which is both patient- and technique-dependent. It is the authors' opinion that any periorbital HA injections to restore contour should be 'under-corrected' to allow for the hydrophilic properties of the filler to complete the correction over time. Blending of the HA in a 50/50 composition with either lidocaine (1 or 2%) or sterile saline can be considered to 'hydrate' the filler, thereby giving it the 'water it seeks' to minimize post-injection swelling. This can be equated to injecting an expanded wet sponge instead of a dry sponge. At the very least, minimal amounts of HA should be injected to avoid the necessity of 'melting' swollen blue-tinged product (Tyndall effect) months later. Hyaluronidase reversal of excess product is effective but inevitably results in prolonged (one week) visible oedema of the region with its associated anxiety for patient and physician.

Again it must be emphasized that periorbital injection therapy should be based on a sound understanding of the anatomy of the region to avoid immediate and delayed adverse events.

The biophysical properties of the selected product (thin with easy spreadability) and the anatomy of the region (injecting above or below the active orbicularis muscle) will indeed dictate the eventual result. Furthermore, the injection technique selected can help with the issue of dark circles commonly seen infraorbitally. These latter result from a combination of factors that include excess pigment, shadowing due to the concavity, and Tyndall effect of the blood vessels of the region through thin skin. Correcting the contour (removing the shadow) and covering the vessels with a thin layer of product (hiding the deep Tyndall effect) can therefore lead to a desirable lightening effect of the region (Figure 5.18).

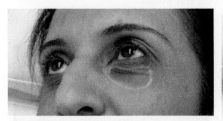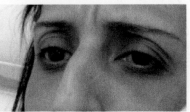

Figure 5.18 Immediate lightening of infraorbital dark circles after subdermal placement of a thin hyaluronic acid filler (see text).

5.6.1 Treatment of the Tear Trough (Medial Canthus to Medial Iris)

The particular anatomy of the orbicularis muscle, as noted above, suggests that tear trough (medial canthus to medial iris) *deep filling* by cannula or needle must be limited to small volumes (<0.1 cm³) (Figure 5.19). This is because deposition of the product is intramuscular and subject to eventual 'balling up' (like a toothpaste tube squeezed from the middle) due to the repeated contractions of squinting and blinking. For deep tear troughs, this means that adequate correction involves a bilayered approach [34], placing small quantities both deep and above the muscle (see later), allowing for freedom of muscle movement (Figure 5.20). When performing a deep correction of the tear trough groove, due to the proximity of the angular artery and vein, the authors prefer to deposit the product in the 'safer' location *on* the infraorbital rim and no further medial than the inner limbus of the iris. Great care must be taken not to inject any HA behind the orbital septum anywhere along the infraorbital rim, as this can lead to prolonged recurrent bouts of periorbital swelling. Instillation of product should be carried out 3–4 mm below the upper margin of the infraorbital rim as the orbital septum has been noted in many cadaver dissections to extend 2–3 mm below the palpable superior edge. The treatment can be performed by direct vertical needle puncture, or preferably via a lateral approach with a cannula, followed by milking of the product into the more hazardous medial trough with the thumb or forefinger. Again,

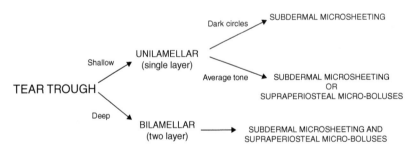

Figure 5.19 Algorithm for the treatment of the tear trough.

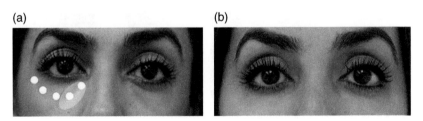

Figure 5.20 (a) Treatment of the tear trough and infraorbital hollow (see text); (b) result at one year.

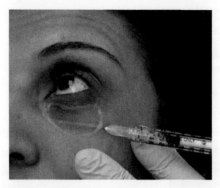

Figure 5.21 Superficial subdermal injection of minute quantities of blended HA filler in the subpalpebral region using a 30G cannula.

for this deeper injection technique, it is recommended to inject no more than 0.05 cm³ of minimal viscosity filler that spreads easily. The solo deep injection technique is often quite adequate in correcting mild tear trough depressions where dark discolouration is not significant.

When dark circles and a mild tear trough depression is present, the preferred technique is to place a very thin layer of thin or hydrated HA subdermally with a needle or cannula [35]. The plane is easily found above the muscle by flattening the angle of the cannula to parallel the skin surface once introduced laterally through the hole of the needle port (Figure 5.21). A very thin sheet of product is fanned over the orbicularis muscle, helping to obscure the Tyndall effect of the underlying plexus of vessels, thereby lightening the region. This technique is very rewarding, but can be technically challenging in delivering the 'microdroplets' necessary to avoid visibility and palpability. An important injection tip is to place the plunger of the syringe in the palm or at the base of the thumb and to deliver the product by gently squeezing.

5.6.2 Treatment of the Lateral Infraorbital Crescent and Lateral Canthus

More laterally in the infraorbital region, filler placement on bone into the SOOF under the orbicularis is ideal for infraorbital rim contouring and camouflage, allowing for unrestricted action of the overlying muscle (Figure 5.22). Again a modicum of product (preferably blended) should be instilled (<0.2 cm³) by mini-bolus needle or cannula to allow for future hydrophilic expansion. Superficial layering of product can also be done with cannula while simultaneously subcising deep static adhering crow's feet from the underlying muscle (Figures 5.20 and 5.23). A novel approach employed for the past two years by one of the authors (AS) involves adding botulinum toxin to

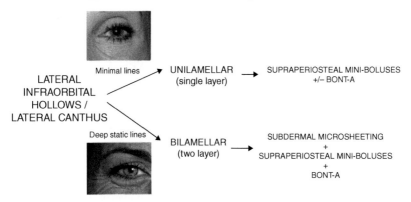

Figure 5.22 Algorithm for the treatment of the lateral infraorbital hollows and lateral canthus.

(a)   (b)

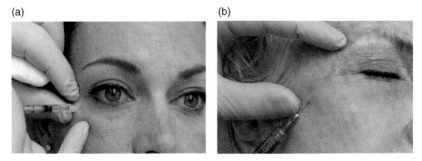

Figure 5.23 Treatment of the lateral infraorbital/canthal region by microbolus vertical 31G needle puncture (a) and/or cannula (b) (see text).

(a)   (b)

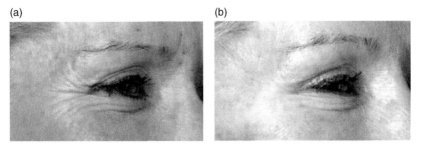

Figure 5.24 'Mesomix' (see text) treatment of crow's feet before (a) and one year after (b) the procedure.

the blended filler ('mesomix') with the subdermal cannula approach, thereby delivering both products into the same desired plane. Preliminary results of this technique (submitted for publication) have shown duration of improvement in crow's feet lasting beyond 18 months (Figure 5.24).

Treatment of the lateral canthus with filler is often overlooked by injection therapists and offers a rejuvenative effect in recreating the youthful lateral canthal 5–10° upward tilt. This is commonly achieved by a supraperiosteal bolus (0.05–0.1 cm³ of a moderate G′ HA) by vertical puncture with needle or by deposition with cannula (Figure 5.25).

5.6.3 Treatment of the Nasojugal Groove

Treatment of the nasojugal groove (lid–cheek junction lateral to the tear trough) extending down on the cheek can be frustrating for the injector due to the tethering effect of the underlying orbito-malar ligament (Figure 5.26). Usually, reasonable correction can be achieved through a multilayer structured approach of placing small pillars of stiffer product on bone, followed by layering of intermediate G′ product subcutaneously and thinner product subdermally. Several sessions of conservative treatment spaced several months apart may be necessary to achieve desirable results (Figure 5.27).

(a)   (b)

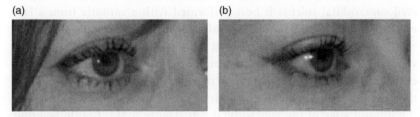

Figure 5.25 Treatment of the lateral canthus before (a) and six months after (b), producing a 5–10° lateral upward canthal tilt.

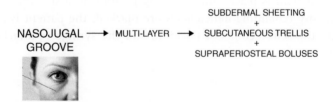

Figure 5.26 Algorithm for the treatment of the nasojugal groove.

(a)   (b)

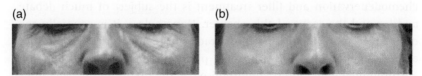

Figure 5.27 Treatment of the nasojugal groove before (a), and one year after (b), using the multilayer technique (see text).

(a) (b) (c)

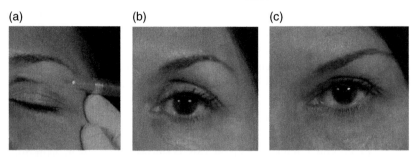

Figure 5.28 (a) Treatment of the infrabrow region with cannula – the cannula is lifted to show the depth of injection; (b) the A-frame deformity before treatment; (c) the result immediately after 0.15 cm³ of blended HA.

5.6.4 Treatment of the Infrabrow Hollow

Treatment of the infrabrow hollow (A-frame deformity or exaggerated supraorbital sulcus) is best performed with a cannula from a lateral approach overlying the lateral supraorbital rim, the cantilever effect of which protects inadvertent damage to the globe [15]. As for superficial injections to the tear trough, the cannula is flattened upon entry into the subdermal plane and passes with little resistance towards the superior medial canthus superficial to the orbicularis muscle along the inferior edge of the supraorbital rim (Figure 5.28). Gentle layering of thin blended HA can be performed, avoiding the supraorbital and supratrochlear neurovascular bundles that exit the orbital cavity more superiorly. The syringe can be unhooked leaving the cannula in situ while the patient is placed into a sitting position to assess the created contour. Any remaining deficiencies are marked, the patient is placed back into the semirecumbent position, and the syringe re-attached to complete the treatment.

5.6.5 Combination with Other Treatments

The periorbital region is often synergistically treated with combination treatments to yield the best results. Timing and treatment syntax of chemodenervation and filler treatment is the subject of much debate, and beyond the scope of this chapter. Nonetheless, it is generally recommended to avoid treating the infraorbital region with both products at the same session due to possible prolonged oedema resulting from HA-prompted fluid ingress compromised by the toxin-diminished pumping action of the muscle and lymphatics [36]. Contrary to prelaser toxin treatment to improve results, skin resurfacing procedures of the periorbital region are probably better managed when performed weeks before any filler placement.

5.7 Conclusion

Periorbital rejuvenation using injectable fillers can create outstanding clinical results and in properly selected cases provides practitioners with non-surgical treatment options (Figures 5.29–5.32). Both cannula and

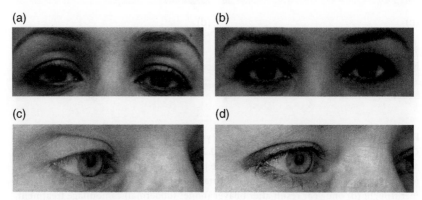

Figure 5.29 (a) Typical pattern of pan-volume loss of the infrabrow region in a Persian patient: (b) one year after 0.2 cm³ of blended HA; (c) asymmetric infrabrow/upper lid region in a Caucasian patient; (d) one year after 0.1 cm³ of blended HA.

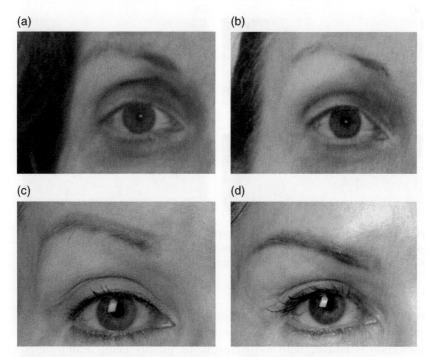

Figure 5.30 (a) Orbital hollowing in a patient with 'coup de sabre' from linear sclero-derma; (b) one year after 0.25 cm³ of blended HA; (c) the peaked brow developed in a patient after botulinum toxin (BoNT-A) treatment reveals infrabrow volume depletion; (d) one month result after BoNT-A correction of brow height and 0.2 cm³ of blended HA to the infrabrow.

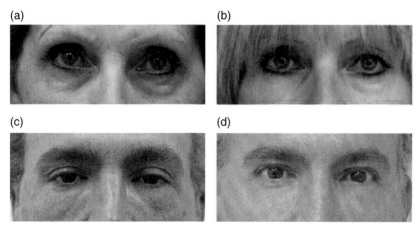

Figure 5.31 (a) Infraorbital crescents and 'eyebags' in a surgery-averse 62-year-old Caucasian female; (b) one year result after 0.2 cm³ of blended HA; (c) tear troughs and nasojugal grooves in a 55-year-old male patient with previous visible fat/poly-methyl methacrylate injections to the subcutaneous layer of the medial cheek and tear trough; (d) one year result after bilayer (bone; subdermal) camouflage treatment with blended HA.

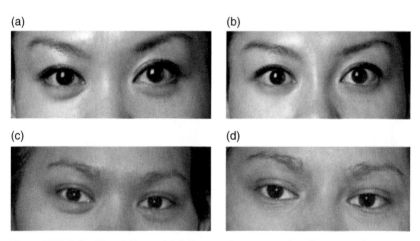

Figure 5.32 Infraciliary fullness: (a) 'baby eyes' in a Korean female patient; (b) one year after bilayer treatment with 0.15 cm³ blended HA; (c) 'worm eyes' in a female Chinese patient; (d) one year after bilayer treatment with 0.1 cm³ blended HA.

needle injection techniques are efficacious in providing good or optimal results for most patients [37]. It must be stressed that avoiding over-correction is crucial, with most treatments usually being administered over two sessions, depending upon individual patient characteristics and requirements. The goal is to create a beautiful youthful periorbital complex that exhibits gentle convexities, smooth transitions from eyelids to surrounding tissues, adequate volume that softens underlying bony margins, and provides for an overall refreshed look. The high mobility and thin skin of the region require a proper selection of limited product of appropriate 'personality' deployed with a 'light touch', the combination of which can dramatically improve a tired look. The duration of effect is typically prolonged, with significant benefits observed beyond 12 months.

References

1. Levy, J., Foulsham, T., and Kingstone, A. (2013). Monsters are people too. *Biol. Lett.* 9: 20120850.
2. Du, S., Tao, Y., and Martinez, A.M. (2014 Apr). Compound facial expressions of emotion. *Proc. Natl. Acad. Sci.* 111 (15): 1454–1462.
3. Wong, C.H., Hsieh, M.K., and Mendelson, B. (2012 Jun). The tear trough ligament: anatomical basis for the tear trough deformity. *Plast. Reconstr. Surg.* 129 (6): 1392–1402.
4. Ghavami, A., Pessa, J.E. et al. (2008 Mar). The orbicularis retaining ligament of the medial orbit: closing the circle. *Plast. Reconstr. Surg.* 121 (3): 994–1001.
5. Rohrich, R.J., Arbique, G.M., Wong, C. et al. (2009 Sep). The anatomy of subocularis fat: implications for periorbital rejuvenation. *Plast. Reconstr. Surg.* 124 (3): 946–951.
6. Ercikti, N., Apaydin, N., and Kirici, Y. (2017 Jan). Location of the infraorbital foramen with reference to soft tissue landmarks. *Surg. Radiol. Anat.* 39 (1): 11–15.
7. Coleman, S.R. and Grover, R. (2006 Jan-Feb). The anatomy of the aging face: volume loss and changes in 3-dimensional topography. *Aesthet. Surg. J.* 26 (1): S4–S9.
8. Lambros, V. (2007 Oct). Observations on periorbital and midface aging. *Plast. Reconstr. Surg.* 120 (5): 1367–1376.
9. Fitzgerald, R. and Vleggaar, D. (2011 Jan-Feb). Facial volume restoration of the ageing face with poly-l-lactic acid. *Dermatol. Ther.* 24 (1): 2–27.
10. Pessa, J.E., Desvigne, L.D., Lambros, V.S. et al. (1999 Sep-Oct). Changes in ocular globe-to-orbital rim position with age: implications for aesthetic blepharoplasty of the lower eyelids. *Aesthet. Plast. Surg.* 23 (5): 337–342.
11. Chen, Y.S., Tsai, T.H., Wu, M.L. et al. (2008 Oct). Evaluation of age-related intraorbital fat herniation through computed tomography. *Plast. Reconstr. Surg.* 122 (4): 1191–1198.
12. Camirand, A., Doucet, J., and Harris, J. (1997 Nov). Anatomy, pathophysiology, and prevention of senile enophthalmia and associated herniated lower eyelid fat pads. *Plast. Reconstr. Surg.* 100 (6): 1535–1546.
13. Ahmadi, H., Shams, P.N., Davies, N. et al. (2007 Mar). Age-related changes in the normal sagittal relationship between globe and orbit. *J. Plast. Reconstr. Aesthet. Surg.* 60 (3): 246–250.
14. Kpodzo, D.S., Nahai, F., and McCord, C. (2014 Feb). Malar mounds and festoons: review of current management. *Aesthet. Surg. J.* 34 (2): 235–248.
15. Liew, S. and Nguyen, D.Q. (2011 Jun). Nonsurgical volumetric upper periorbital rejuvenation: a plastic surgeon's perspective. *Aesthet. Plast. Surg.* 35 (3): 319–325.
16. Camp, M., Wong, W. et al. (2011 Feb). A quantitative analysis of periorbital aging with three-dimensional surface imaging. *J. Plast. Reconstr. Aesthet. Surg.* 64 (2): 148–154.

17. Papageorgiou, K.I., Mancini, R. et al. (2012 Jan). A three-dimensional construct of the aging eyebrow: the illusion of volume loss. *Aesthet. Surg. J.* 32 (1): 46–57.
18. Israel, H. (1977 Jul). The dichotomous pattern of craniofacial expansion during aging. *Am. J. Phys. Anthropol.* 47 (1): 47–51.
19. Forsberg, C.M., Eliasson, S., and Westergren, H. (1991 Aug). Face height and tooth eruption in adults – a 20-year follow-up investigation. *Eur. J. Orthod.* 13 (4): 249–254.
20. Bondevik, O. (1995 Dec). Growth changes in the cranial base and the face: a longitudinal cephalometric study of linear and angular changes in adult Norwegians. *Eur. J. Orthod.* 17 (6): 525–532.
21. West, K.S. and McNamara, J.A. Jr. (1999 May). Changes in the craniofacial complex from adolescence to midadulthod: a cephalometric study. *Am. J. Orthod. Dentofac. Orthop.* 115 (5): 521–532.
22. Akgul, A.A. and Toygar, T.U. (2002 Nov). Natural craniofacial changes in the third decade of life: a longtidinal study. *Am. J. Orthod. Dentofac. Orthop.* 122 (5): 512–522.
23. Pecora, N.G., Baccetti, T., and McNamara, J.A. Jr. (2008 Oct). The aging craniofacial complex: a longitudinal cephalometric study from late adolescence to late adulthood. *Am. J. Orthod. Dentofac. Orthop.* 134 (4): 496–505.
24. Albert, A., Ricanek, K. Jr., and Patterson, E. (2007 Oct). A review of the literature on the aging skull and face: implications for forensic science research and applications. *Forensic Sci. Int.* 172 (1): 1–9.
25. Shaw, R.B. Jr. and Kahn, D.M. (2007 Feb). Aging of the midface bony elements: a three-dimensional computed tomographic study. *Plast. Reconstr. Surg.* 119 (2): 675–681.
26. Odunze, M., Rosenberg, D.S., and Few, J.W. (2008 Mar). Periorbital aging and ethnic considerations: a focus on the lateral canthal complex. *Plast. Reconstr. Surg.* 121 (3): 1002–1008.
27. Raspaldo, H., Bettens, R., and Giordano, P.H. (2006). Midface enhancement: anatomy and techniques. In: *Facial Plastic and Reconstructive Surgery* (ed. H.D. Vuyk and P.J. Lohuis), 105–122. New York: Oxford University Press.
28. Rohrich, R.J., Pessa, J.E., and Ristow, B. (2008Jun). The youthful cheek and the deep medial fat compartment. *Plast. Reconstr. Surg.* 121 (6): 2107–2112.
29. Raspaldo, H., Aziza, R., Belhaouari, L. et al. (2011 Feb). How to achieve synergy between volume replacement and filling products for global facial rejuvenation. *J Cosmet Laser Ther* 13: 77–86.
30. Fagien, S. and Raspaldo, H. (2007). Facial rejuvenation with botulinum neurotoxin: an anatomical and experiential perspective. *J. Cosmet. Laser Ther.* 9 (Suppl 1): 23–31.
31. Raspaldo, H., Baspeyras, M., Bellity, P. et al. (Consensus Group)(2011 Mar). Upper- and mid-face anti-aging treatment and prevention using onabotulinumtoxin a: the 2010 multidisciplinary French consensus – part 1. *J. Cosmet. Dermatol.* 10 (1): 36–50.
32. Raspaldo, H. (2008 Sep). Volumizing effect of a new hyaluronic acid sub-dermal facial filler: a retrospective analysis based on 102 cases. *J Cosmet Laser Ther* 10 (3): 134–142.
33. Swift, A. and Remington, K. (2011 Jul). BeautiPHIcation™: a global approach to facial beauty. *Clin. Plast. Surg.* 38 (3): 347–377.
34. Kane, M.A. (2005 Sep-Oct). Commentary on filling the periorbital hollows with hyaluronic acid gel: initial experience with 244 injections. *Ophthal. Plast. Reconstr. Surg.* 22 (5): 341–343.
35. Kane, M.A. (2005 Sep-Oct). Treatment of tear trough deformity and lower lid bowing with injectable hyaluronic acid. *Aesthet. Plast. Surg.* 29 (5): 363–367.

36. Sundaram, H., Liew, S. et al. (2016 May). Global aesthetics consensus: hyaluronic acid fillers and botulinum toxin type a – recommendations for combined treatment and optimizing outcomes in diverse patient populations. *Plast. Reconstr. Surg.* 137 (5): 1410–1423.
37. Raspaldo, H. (24–28 September 2008). *New era of facial-3D rejuvenation using injectable products and how to measure the results.* Annual Conference in the 31st year of the European Academy of Facial Plastic Surgery, Düsseldorf, Germany. Bologna, Italy: Medimond S.r.l.

CHAPTER 6

The Midface and Cheeks

Jeanette M. Black, Ardalan Minokadeh and Derek H. Jones
Skin Care and Laser Physicians of Beverly Hills, Los Angeles, CA, USA

6.1 Background

It is difficult to objectively identify what makes someone beautiful, yet regardless of ethnic background, age, or nationality, people universally share a sense of what is attractive [1]. Of the objective things that people identify as beautiful, facial shape plays a vital role [1]. The midface and cheeks are a fundamental component of facial shape and this area loses volume with senescence due to malar bone reabsorption and the atrophy of midface fat pads [2–4]. Cheek augmentation with injectable fillers has been shown to improve how patients feel about their own attractiveness [5]. It is essential that the injector have an in-depth understanding of beauty, and be well studied in the art of facial proportions and relationships [1]. The loss of bony support and lipoatrophy of the midface can lead to the descent of soft tissues, creating lower face laxity and folds which may be improved by volumizing the upper face [6]. Given that correction of the midface and cheek can improve the appearance of surrounding facial structures, volumization of the midface and cheeks is often one of the first treatments to consider when evaluating a patient.

6.2 Age-related Lipoatrophy of the Midface and Cheeks

The most common cause of facial lipoatrophy is age-related, where volume loss in the midface and cheeks affects the surrounding structures, including the tear troughs and the lower face [4, 6]. Correcting the volume

Injectable Fillers: Facial Shaping and Contouring, Second Edition.
Edited by Derek H. Jones and Arthur Swift.
© 2019 John Wiley & Sons Ltd. Published 2019 by John Wiley & Sons Ltd.
Companion website: www.wiley.com/go/jones/injectable_fillers

deficit in the midface has been shown to reduce the depth of nasolabial folds [6]. Alterations in the midface include volume loss from both hard and soft tissues, which result in midfacial hollowing, demarcation of the cosmetic units, and a gaunt appearance. The underlying geometric alterations of distinct facial adipose compartments contributes significantly to the changes of the ageing face [7]. Understanding the facial adipose system and its age-related changes allows for optimal injectable volume restoration [8]. Additionally, volumizing the midface and cheeks appropriately can lead to an improvement of the global aesthetic appearance [6].

Facial ageing is a complex synergy of skin textural and elastotic changes, muscular hyperactivity, and fat dysmorphism, and the resulting volume deficit of the midface produces a less youthful and attractive appearance [7]. To help objectify the changes in the midface, the midface volume deficit scale (MFVDS) was developed and used in the pivotal Juvederm Voluma® XC trial [9]. The MFVDS is a validated six-point photometric scale, which evaluates the degree of concavity in the zygomaticomalar region, anteromedial cheek, and submalar region [9]. The scale also evaluates the degree of tear trough and nasolabial development, the degree of nasojugal folds and prejowl sulcus formation, the prominence of bony landmarks, and the visibility of underlying musculature [9]. This scale can be used to help quantify the degree of deficit and can help the injector estimate the amount of volume needed for optimal correction.

6.3 HIV Lipoatrophy

Special consideration should be made for patients with HIV lipoatrophy associated with the use of highly active antiretroviral therapy (HAART) [10, 11]. HIV facial lipoatrophy is characterized by facial volume loss that affects the contours of the temples and orbits as well as the midface and cheeks [10]. This condition is socially stigmatizing, impacts patients' adherence to HAART, psychological health, career, and quality of life including feelings of distress, depression, anxiety, and social isolation [10]. HIV lipoatrophy of the midface and cheek can be particularly recognizable. Correction of this lipoatrophy is linked to improvement in the quality of life in patients in categories including health perception, mental health, social function, and emotional status [10]. The Carruthers Lipoatrophy Severity Scale is often used as a standardized measurement to assess the degree of lipoatrophy and can help estimate the amount of volume replacement needed [10]. Sculptra® (poly-L-lactic acid) and Radiesse® (calcium hydroxylapatite) are both FDA approved for the treatment of HIV lipoatrophy and have been commonly used for this condition [10]. The authors have found that treatment using highly purified 1000-cSt

(a)   (b)

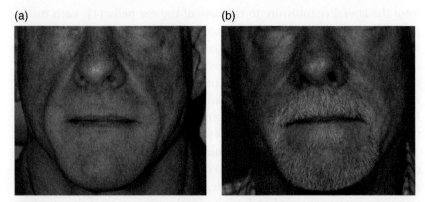

Figure 6.1 Patient before (a) and 11 years after (b) treatment with highly purified liquid injectable silicone for HIV associated facial lipoatrophy.

silicone oil with a microdroplet serial puncture technique has been particularly helpful for these HIV patients who often require large quantities of long lasting or permanent volumization [11, 12]. Highly purified silicone oil has proven to be effective in our experience, although a small percentage may develop late-appearing firmness, nodule or overcorrection that is treatable with 5-fluorouracil admixed with triamcinolone. [11, 12] (Figure 6.1). As a non-permanent option for HIV lipoatrophy of the midface, we have found 20 mg ml^{-1} hyaluronic acid filler (Juvederm Voluma XC) useful. Indeed, the long-term improvement using this filler, lasting for at least three years in one patient, has been published from our group [13]. Autologous fat transfer, polyacrylamide gel, and polymethylmethacrylate (PMMA) have been used to treat HIV lipoatrophy with variable outcomes and generally we do not recommend these treatments [10]. Treatment of HIV facial lipoatrophy with polyalkylimide gel has been associated with late appearing abscesses, and we consider it contraindicated for facial volumizing (see Chapter 11).

6.4 Treatment Planning

At the initial consultation it important to take a thorough history and ask about any previous injectable fillers, permanent implants, surgeries, and/or trauma to the treatment area [2]. It is also helpful to advise patients to abstain from unnecessary medications with anticoagulant properties prior to the procedure, to decrease the risk of swelling and bruising [14]. Any asymmetry should be discussed and documented and all patients should have baseline photographs taken [2]. Treatment plans should be tailored to the anatomic needs of each patient as well as the patient's gender [1]. The ideal female cheek is ovoid and not circular and the cheek axis is angled from the lateral commissure to the base of the ear helix [1]. Each malar prominence has a defined apex, located high on the midface, inferior and lateral to the lateral canthus, and eccentrically located within the cheek oval [1]. The ideal male cheek has less anteromedial fullness with a more subtle, broader, and medial malar prominence [1]. It is important to take these differences into consideration when planning augmentation. Regardless of gender, the malar prominence should not extend higher than the limbus of the lower eyelid [1].

When planning augmentation of midface volume deficit, it is helpful to draw out and measure facial landmarks. Identifying facial landmarks can aid the injector in determining the ideal facial shape for the individual. A technique commonly used to find the ideal prominence of the cheek is to draw Hinderer's Lines. Dr Ulrich Hinderer was a plastic surgeon who developed silicone malar shell implants to correct midface volume deficit in 1975 [4]. He found the best cosmetic outcomes when cheek implants were placed in the upper-outer quadrant of these lines and would draw them to help pinpoint the ideal location for his implants [4]. These lines include a vertical line drawn from the lateral canthus to the oral commissure and an intersecting line marked from the tragus to the nasal ala [4, 15]. The upper outer quadrant of this intersection is targeted for volumization [15] (Figure 6.2). Using Hinderer's Lines can help the injector identify the ideal malar prominence, and respecting these lines can help to assure the appropriate locations are treated without over volumization.

Although a youthful structure is typified by a triangular shape with a full and wide midface, proportion is paramount and great care should be taken to avoid overvolumization [1]. It has been proposed that the 'phi facial width proportion' is the ideal proportion of the midface, in which the

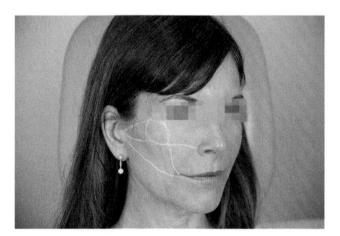

Figure 6.2 Hinderer's Lines. The oval represents the apex of volume of a beautiful female cheek.

distance from one medial canthus to the other medial canthus measures 'x' and the medial canthus to ipsilateral cheek apex measures 1.618× [1] (see Chapter 2). Callipers can be used to measure this ratio when analysing patients [1]. Other mechanisms of treatment planning have been proposed, including placing silicone implant analogues on top of the skin and tracing out these shapes. This technique may help the injector and the patient visualize the planned volumization strategy [16]. 3-D technology may also be used to help simulate treatment plans.

6.5 Injection Techniques and Safety Considerations

Knowledge of the underlying anatomy of the midface and cheek is fundamental for the injector. A basic understanding of the midface vasculature can help decrease the risk of hematoma and the potential for vascular occlusion [17, 18]. The vasculature in the midface includes the facial artery, the angular artery, and the infraorbital artery [17, 18] (Figure 6.3). Given the significant vascular network of the midface and the potential for complications, the authors advise using a blunt tipped cannula when injecting the midface and cheeks, especially when injection is needed in the mid-cheek area medial to the mid-pupillary line (Video 6.1). There are many proposed injection techniques in the midface and cheeks, such as serial puncture depot injections along the zygoma, linear threading, fanning, or cross-hatching. In addition to decreasing the risk of vascular occlusion, the authors find that the use of cannulae in lieu of sharp needles helps the

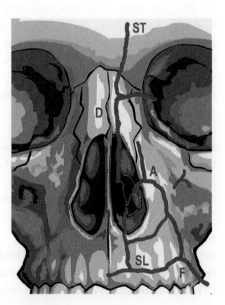

Figure 6.3 Arteries of the midface include the [F]facial artery, [A] angular artery, and the infraorbital artery. Note anastomoses with the [SL] superior labial artery, [DL] dorsal nasal artery and [ST] supratrochlear artery.

injector more precisely volumize the midface and cheek, with a reduction of swelling and bruising after treatments.

6.6 Filling Agents

Various filler products have been used to correct midface volume deficit and enhance cheeks. The ideal filler is safe, long lasting, and has a high G' or high cohesivity to maximize the lifting capacity of the overlying tissue. Fillers with inherent biostimulatory properties to induce neocollagenesis could potentially increase the longevity of treatments [8]. Although Juvederm Voluma XC and Restylane® Lyft are the only FDA approved filling agents to volumize the midface and cheeks, a variety of products have been used to treat this area [4].

6.6.1 Juvederm Voluma XC

Juvederm Voluma XC (VYC-20L)is a 20 mg ml^{-1} hyaluronic acid volumizing filler with 0.3% lidocaine, which was the first injectable filler specifically FDA approved for age-related midface volume deficit [4, 19]. The pivotal study was a multicentre, single-blind, randomized controlled trial which showed good safety profiles and excellent outcomes for up to two years [9]. It is an ideal filler because it is biodegradable, reversible, and has significant lifting capacity [4, 9, 20]. It has a mixture of low and high molecular weight hyaluronic acid and a higher cross-linking ratio [4, 20]. This results in increased cohesivity and viscosity, allowing for retention of structure after deep injection, and a higher lift capacity than other hyaluronic acid fillers [4, 9]. The product is indicated for subcutaneous or supraperiosteal injection for facial volumizing and contouring [4]. Repeat treatments over 12–24 months with Juvederm Voluma XC has been shown to be well tolerated and results in high levels of effectiveness and patient satisfaction [19]. Treatment sites for Juvederm Voluma XC have been divided into three subregions: the zygomaticulomalar, anteromedial cheek, and submalar [21] (Figure 6.4). All three of the treatment regions have been shown to be safe and provide high patient satisfaction [21] (Figures 6.5–6.7). Injection of the midface should adhere to the principles and mathematics of facial beauty (see Chapter 2). Juvederm Voluma XC has proven to be reversible in vivo with hyaluronidase [22].

6.6.2 Restylane Lyft

Restylane Lyft, formerly known as Perlane® (LGP-HA-L), is a 20 mg ml^{-1} large gel particle hyaluronic acid volumizing filler with 0.3% lidocaine [23]. The effectiveness of Perlane in volumizing the midface was evaluated

Mid-Face Treatment Areas

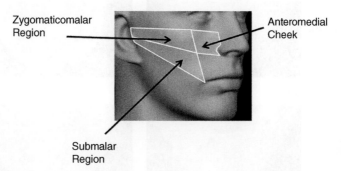

Figure 6.4 Treatment sites for Juvederm Voluma XC include zygomaticomalar, anteromedial cheek, and submalar.

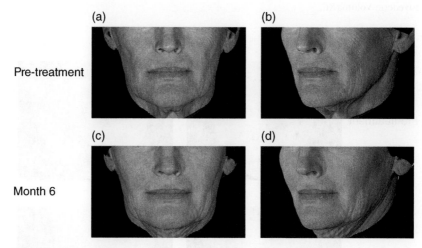

Figure 6.5 Patient before (a and b) and six months after (c and d) treatment with Juvederm Voluma XC.

in an open-label Canadian study [23]. This was a 24-week trial which included 40 patients [23]. At week 24 there was continued improvement noted in 90% of patients as rated by evaluators and in 82.5% of patients as rated by the subjects [23]. The study also demonstrated a good safety profile within the 24 weeks [23]. Similar to Juvederm Voluma XC, this hyaluronic acid product is biodegradable, reversible, and also provides adequate lifting capacity. Restylane Lyft is FDA approved to correct age-related volume loss in the cheek area. The pivotal trial was a 12-month study with 200 patients at 12 centres, showing efficacy and safety for this treatment indication [24]. In the trial, a significantly greater

(a)   (b)

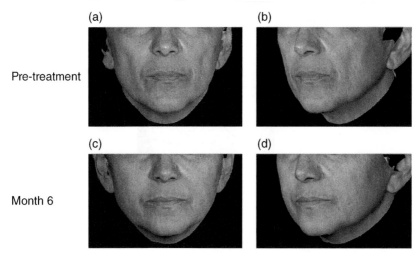

Pre-treatment

Month 6

Figure 6.6 Patient before (a and b) and six months after (c and d) treatment with Juvederm Voluma XC.

(a)   (b)

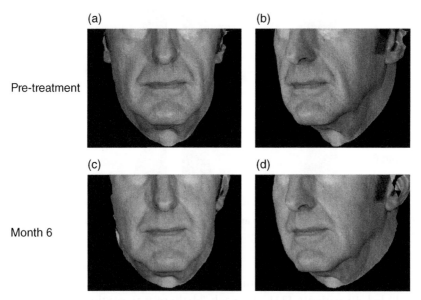

Pre-treatment

Month 6

(c)   (d)

Figure 6.7 Patient before (a and b) and six months after (c and d) treatment with Juvederm Voluma XC.

percentage of subjects achieved treatment success through month 12 as compared with subjects without treatment [24]. Treatment success was defined as at least 1-grade improvement on the Medicis Midface Volume Scale (MMVS) [24]. Additionally, 85% of subjects maintained global aesthetic improvement at one year after initial treatment [24].

6.6.3 Radiesse

Radiesse (calcium hydroxylapatite (CaHA)) is a biocompatible injectable filler that is FDA approved for subdermal implantation to treat moderate to severe facial wrinkles and folds, such as nasolabial folds, the restoration of HIV facial lipoatrophy, and subdermal implantation for hand augmentation. Although not FDA approved for cheek augmentation other than for the correction of HIV facial lipoatrophy, the product is commonly used subcutaneously or periosteally for midface and cheek voluminization [4] (Figures 6.8 and 6.9, and Video 6.2). CaHA is visible on radiography, but does not obscure underlying structures or pathology [25]. The product works well in the midface given it's high lift capacity, and results usually persist for about a year or longer [4]. A recent report documented a patient with sustained visible tissue volume in the midface 2.5 years after malar injection of CaHA, although the product was no longer visible on MRI images, indicating a collagen-stimulating effect [25]. Unlike the

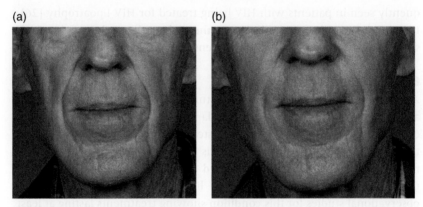

(a)   (b)

Figure 6.8 Patient before (a) and after (b) treatment with Radiesse for age-related lipoatrophy.

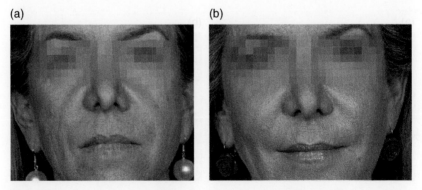

(a)   (b)

Figure 6.9 Patient before (a) and after (b) treatment with Radiesse for age-related lipoatrophy.

hyaluronic acid alternatives, CaHA is not reversible with hyaluronidase, and inappropriate placement of product may be unforgiving [26]; when injection is too superficial, persistent lumps can result [26].

6.6.4 Sculptra®
Sculptra (poly-L-lactic acid (PLLA)) consists of lyophilized crystals of PLLA rehydrated with the addition of sterile water 24 hours prior to injection [4]. This biodegradable synthetic polymer stimulates collagen production by causing foreign body reaction and dermal fibrosis [4]. A series of subdermal injections are typically performed over several sessions at six-week intervals and results can take months to achieve [4]. The product is FDA approved to treat facial wrinkles and folds, such as nasolabial folds, and the restoration of HIV lipoatrophy. Although not FDA approved for the treatment of the midface and cheeks, other than to treat HIV lipoatrophy, this product has been commonly used in the area (Figure 6.10). Injection site nodules have been reported with PLLA and these nodules are most frequently seen in patients with HIV being treated for HIV lipoatrophy [26]. Increasing the volume of dilution of the vials with sterile water ($\geq 5\,ml^3$ sterile water, with $1\,ml^3$ lidocaine) lessens the likelihood of nodules [26].

6.6.5 Autologous Fat Transfer
Autologous fat can be harvested with tumescent liposuction, centrifuged, and injected pan-facially with a cannula for volumization [27]. The autologous fat can be placed in small periosteal aliquots in the cheek area and threaded in the midface area [27]. This technique has provided effective results for the treatment of age-related lipoatrophy [27]. Autologous fat transfer has also been used with HIV lipoatrophy and there have been observational studies for this condition showing treatments lasting at least one year and up to four years in one study [10]. This method seems to offer significant volumization and long lasting results; however, duration

(a)   (b)

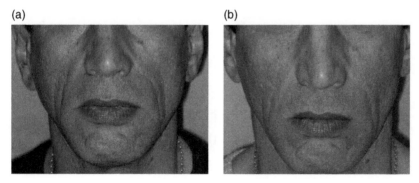

Figure 6.10 Patient before (a) and after (b) treatment with Sculptra for age-related lipoatrophy.

of correction may be highly variable and the necessity of surgical liposuction harvesting limits its popularity.

6.6.6 Silicone

Silikon-1000® is highly purified silicone oil FDA approved for the treatment of retinal detachment, but may be injected off-label for soft tissue augmentation. This permanent filler agent is typically injected using a microdroplet serial puncture technique [11]. The authors have found this product to be particularly useful for the correction of HIV-associated lipoatrophy [11, 12]. The product is injected in limited volumes of 2 ml or less in a series of at least monthly intervals until optimal correction is achieved [11, 12]. Permanent fillers may be associated with a higher incidence of adverse events, and knowledge and experience are key to good outcomes.

6.7 Conclusions

Given the appropriate patient selection and injection technique, a knowledgeable aesthetic physician can effectively enhance a patient's perceived beauty by correcting midface volume deficit. Midface volume deficit can be a result of age-related changes or medical conditions such as HIV lipoatrophy. Injectable procedures in the midface and cheeks are becoming increasingly popular as novel injectable filler products become available. It is critical that the injector respects the underling anatomy of the midface to avoid complications and to provide patients with the best possible outcome.

References

1. Swift, A. (2010). The mathematics of facial beauty: a cheek enhancement guide for the aesthetic injector. In: *Injectable Fillers: Principles and Practice* (ed. D. Jones), 140–157. Oxford, UK: Wiley-Blackwell.
2. Fabi, S. and Goldman, M. (2015). Soft tissue augmentation with hyaluronic acid and calcium hydroxylapatite fillers. In: *Rejuvenation of the Aging Face* (ed. A. Karam and M. Goldman), 15–25. London, UK: JP Medical Ltd.
3. Braz, A. and Sakuma, T. (2012). Midface rejuvenation: an innovative technique to restore cheek volume. *Dermatol. Surg.* 38: 118–120.
4. Tan, M. and Kontis, T. (2015). Midface volumization with injectable fillers. *Facial Plast. Surg. Clin. North Am.* 23: 233–242.
5. Taub, A. (2012). Cheek augmentation improves feeling of facial attractiveness. *J. Drugs Dermatol.* 11 (9): 1077–1080.
6. Biesman, B. and Bowe, W. (2015). Effect of midfacial volume augmentation with non animal stablilized hyaluronic acid on the nasolabial fold and global aesthetic appearance. *J Drugs Dermatol.* 14 (9): 943–947.

7. Donofrio, L. (2000). Fat distribution: a morphologic study of the aging face. *Dermatol. Surg.* 26: 1107–1112.

8. Sadick, F., Dorizas, A., Krueger, N., and Nassar, A. (2015). The facial adipose system: its role in facial aging and approaches to volume restoration. *Dermatol. Surg.* 41: S333–S339.

9. Jones, D. and Murphy, D. (2013). Volumizing hyaluronic acid filler for midface volume deficit: 2-year results from a pivotal single-blind randomized controlled study. *Dermatol. Surg.* 39: 1602–1612.

10. Jagdeo, J., Ho, D., Lo, A., and Carruthers, A. (2015). A systemic review of filler agents for aesthetic treatment of HIV facial lipoatrophy. *Dermatol. Surg.* 73: 1040–1054.

11. Jones, D., Carruthers, A., Orentreich, D. et al. (2004). Highly purified 1000-cSt silicone oil for treatment of human immunodeficiency virus-associated facial lipoatrophy: an open pilot trial. *Dermatol. Surg.* 30: 1279–1286.

12. Jones, D.H., Carruthers, A., Brody, H.J. et al. (accepted for publication) Ten-year and beyond follow up after treatment with highly purified liquid injectable silicone for HIV associated facial lipoatrophy: A report of 164 patients Dermatol. Surg.

13. Hausauer, A.K. and Jones, D.H. (2018). Long-term correction of iatrogenic lipoatrophy with volumizing hyaluronic acid filler. *Dermatol. Surg.* 44: S60–S62.

14. Vanman, M., Fabi, S., and Carruthers, J. (2016). Complication in the cosmetic dermatology patient: a review and our experience (Part 1). *Dermatol. Surg.* 42: 1–11.

15. Hinderer, U. (1975). Malar implants for improvement of the facial appearance. *Plast. Reconstr Surg.* 56 (2): 157–165.

16. Niamtu, J. (2008). Accurate and anatomic midface filler injection by using cheek implants as an injection template. *Dermatol. Surg.* 34: 93–96.

17. Beleznay, K., Carruthers, J., Humphrey, S., and Jones, D. (2015). Avoiding and treating blindness from fillers: a review of the world literature. *Dermatol. Surg.* 41: 1097–1117.

18. Pilsl, U., Anderhuber, F., and Rzany, B. (2012). Anatomy of the cheek: implications for soft tissue augmentation. *Dermatol. Surg.* 38: 1254–1262.

19. Baumann, L., Narins, R., Beer, K. et al. (2015). Volumizing hyaluraonic acid filler for midface volume deficit: results after repeat treatment. *Dermatol. Surg.* 41: S284–S292.

20. Callan, P., Goodman, G., Carlisle, I. et al. (2013). Efficacy and safety of hyaluronic acid filler in subjects treated for correction of midface volume deficiency: a 24 month study. *Clin. Cosmet. Investig. Dermatol.* 6: 81–89.

21. Glaser, D., Kenkel, J., Paradkar-Mitragotri, Murphy D. et al. (2015). Duration of effect by injection volume and facial subregion for volumizing hyaluronic acid filler in treating midface volume deficit. *Dermatol. Surg.* 41: 942–949.

22. Shumate, G., Chopra, R., Jones, D. et al. (2018). In-vivo degradation of cross-linked hyaluronic acid fillers by exogenous hyaluronidases. *Dermatol. Surg.* 44 (8): 1075–1083.

23. Bertucci, V., Lin, X., Axord-Gatley, R. et al. (2013). Safety and effectiveness of large gel particle hyaluronic acid with lidocaine for correction of midface volume loss. *Dermatol. Surg.* 39: 1621–1629.

24. Weiss, R., Moradi, A., Bank, D. et al. (2016). Effectiveness and safety of large gel particle hyaluronic acid with lidocaine for correction of midface volume deficit or contour deficiency. *Dermatol. Surg.* 42 (10): 699–709.

25. Pavicic, T. (2015). Complete biodegradable nature of calcium hydroxylapetite after injection for malar enhancement: an MRI study. *Clin Cosmet Investig Dermatol* 9 (8): 19–25.

26. Cohen, J. (2008). Understanding, avoiding, and managing dermal filler complications. *Dermatol. Surg.* 34: S92–S99.

27. Donofrio, L. Structural autologous lipoaugmentation: a pan-facial technique. *Dermatol. Surg.* 26 (12): 1129–1134.

CHAPTER 7

Injection Rhinoplasty – Aesthetic Considerations and the Anatomical Basis for Safe Injection Techniques

Woffles T.L. Wu

Woffles Wu Aesthetic Surgery and Laser Centre, Singapore

7.1 Introduction

Injection rhinoplasty [1–4] has become one of the most frequently performed cosmetic procedures throughout Asia and refers to the non-surgical technique of enhancing or beautifying the nose using injectable fillers delivered through a sharp needle or cannula. It is a satisfying technique for both patient and physician, relatively painless, and the results are visible immediately without patients having to endure a protracted period of swelling, bruising, and recovery. It is also cost effective as significant improvements can be seen with a single syringe of filler. Patients readily accept that they have to return on a regular basis for touch-ups as it is a quick convenient procedure and there is minimal downtime involved. Some of these patients may have an intention to eventually have surgery, using the injection technique as a stepping stone to evaluate the suitability of their new look. For many patients, the injection technique is so convenient and the results more than adequate that they may decide to avoid surgical intervention completely.

The technique is also growing in popularity amongst aesthetic physicians in the West who treat Asian patients or find it convenient to smooth out or correct minor contour irregularities in Caucasian patients without having to resort to surgery.

With a greater knowledge of the underlying nasal anatomy and the development of a variety of new fillers with different degrees of cohesivity, injection rhinoplasty techniques have improved considerably over the past

Injectable Fillers: Facial Shaping and Contouring, Second Edition.
Edited by Derek H. Jones and Arthur Swift.
© 2019 John Wiley & Sons Ltd. Published 2019 by John Wiley & Sons Ltd.
Companion website: www.wiley.com/go/jones/injectable_fillers

15 years. It is now possible to elevate the dorsum, blending it artistically with the medial eyebrow (the orbitonasal line), project the tip forward or tilt it upwards, lower the columella, narrow the nostrils, and change the basal support of the nose by volumizing the premaxilla and the sides of the pyriform aperture, thus profoundly changing the shape and projection of the nose. These more cohesive and stable fillers can be placed where a cartilage graft may have been required and can more closely mimic the result of a surgical rhinoplasty.

Unfortunately, injection rhinoplasty is also a technique that has found favour with beauticians and unlicensed practitioners, which has sometimes caused severe complications. Even amongst well-trained physicians, complications can occur, the most devastatating being vascular occlusions leading to skin necrosis and in some patients, blindness. The best way to minimize these complications is to understand the anatomy of the areas being injected and to practise safe injection technique.

7.1.1 Aesthetic Considerations of Nasal Augmentation

Augmentation of the nose, whether by surgery or by injection, is popular amongst Asians as it addresses one of the key concerns of those seeking aesthetic improvement – a flat nose. The Asian face is typically boxy and wide with a retruded midface marked by inadequate projection of the nose and chin leading to the perception of a flat, squarish face. Shallow orbits contribute to the appearance of bulgy eyeballs which sometimes project beyond the radix of the nose, further contributing to a flat, featureless face. Vertical lengthening and ovalizing of the face together with increased anterior projection of the midface structures such as the forehead, nose and chin are key components of improving facial aesthetics in the Asian face [5, 6].

7.2 Historical Context

The concept of injection rhinoplasty is not new in Asia. For many decades before and after the Second World War, paraffin, wax, and then liquid silicone was used by beauticians and sometimes by doctors to enhance the bridge of the nose without surgery. The typical history given by such patients was that the initial results of the injections were encouraging with the patient returning for more injections to the nose and then venturing further to augment the cheeks, chin, and forehead, believing this technique to be safe and free of long-term complications. However, these permanent fillers often swelled, migrated, or created granulomas and hard encapsulated nodules wherever they were injected or had migrated to. Over time, many of these patients (mostly women) developed a similar dysmorphic facies with a bloated elephantine nose, a witches chin deformity and abnormally puffed up foreheads and cheeks – 'silicone sisters'. Removal of the impregnated permanent material with a restoration to a normal facies was extremely challenging and virtually impossible to achieve. The only area amenable to near total removal and an acceptable aesthetic outcome was in the nose as there are no significant motor nerves that run across it.

With this historical background, it would seem logical not to inject any permanent fillers into the nasal region for fear of similar complications and encountering subsequent difficulty in removing the substance should the patient change their mind and wish to have surgery instead.

Furthermore, the threat of blindness has recently become a major concern for physicians performing this technique [7–17].

7.3 The Anatomical Basis for Safe Injections

As the concept and techniques of facial autologous fat grafts (for all parts of the face, including the nose) and filler injections for non-surgical nasal augmentation have spread globally, so too have the incidence and reporting of serious complications. There are now nearly 100 cases of blindness reported in patients who have had either fat or filler injections to the nose, forehead, and periorbital regions [18]. In all patients, the visual loss was permanent despite any remedial measures being implemented. Of these cases, approximately half were due to fat and the other half due to a variety of synthetic injectable fillers. Surprisingly, over 75% of these complications were associated with the use of a cannula, indicating that its use may not be as safe as we once believed. It is therefore timely to review the anatomy of the nose and its immediate surroundings to understand why these complications occurred and how we can develop safe techniques for injection rhinoplasty.

Wu in 1990 [19] described the presence of five soft tissue layers overlying the osseocartilaginous framework of the nose, namely: the skin envelope (thicker at the tip than over the dorsum or radix), the superficial fibrofatty areolar layer, the middle fibromuscular layer, the deep areolar layer, and periosteum or perichondrium (Figure 7.1a and b).

The nasal skin is thick and firm and difficult to inject. The periosteum and perichondrium are both densely adherent to the underlying osseocartilaginous framework and similarly difficult to inject into or beneath. This leaves a plane of least resistance sandwiched between these two outer and inner layers, made up of the fibromuscular layer and the two areolar layers above and below it. The superficial and deep areolar layers represent two natural planes of dissection that allow either the skin to be easily dissected off the fibromuscular layer, or the fibromuscular layer to be separated from the perichicondrial/periosteal layer. The vascular network of the nose lies on the surface of this fibromuscular layer (Figure 7.2a–d).

(a)

(b)

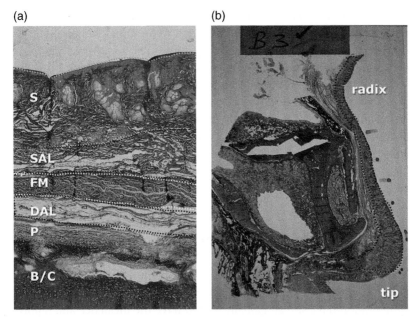

Figure 7.1 (a) Histology of the nose showing the five different soft tissue layers on top of the nasal bone or cartilage (B/C), namely: S, overlying skin (S), superficial areolar layer (SAL), fibromuscular layer (FM), deep areolar layer (DAL), periosteum or perichondrium (P); (b) saggital section of the nose and septum showing the thickness of the nasal skin increases towards the tip.

Figure 7.2 (a–d) Anatomical dissection of the nose and its soft tissue layers. The skin envelope has already been removed (a) and the fibromuscular layer has been split in the midline and reflected to show the underlying osseocartilaginous framework (b). No blood vessels lie beneath the fibromuscular layer. All major blood vessels lie on its superior surface. Therefore, the safest place to inject a filler in the nose is on the bone or periosteum itself or on the dorsal edge of the cartilaginous septum, ensuring that the supratrochlear and supraorbital foramina are first indentified by palpation and protected from the needle point. It is unwise to allow a needle to enter any of the facial bony foramina. Over the nose, the arterial supply [20] is paired on either side with an alar, columellar (derived from the facial artery), and dorsal nasal (a branch of the ophthalmic artery) artery on each side with a vascular watershed in the midline of the nose. The midline of the nose is therefore an anatomically safe place for sharp needle injections which should endeavour to be directly on the underlying bone or cartilage of the nose. (c and d) In these separate specimens, the facial artery is seen coursing upwards through the nasolabial region to the junction of the alar lobule with the lip where it splits into a robust columellar artery which runs in the nostril sill and then along the columella to the tip of the nose and an alar artery, which curves around the alar groove and supplies the alar lobule. An attenuated tributary of the alar artery continues towards the medial canthus of the eye where it anastamoses with the dorsal nasal artery which in turn is a terminal branch of the ophthalmic artery. Note the paired columellar arteries running superficially along the columella to the tip of the nose where they anastamose with the alar plexus which unites branches from the columellar, alar, and dorsal nasal arteries.

The vasculature of the nose is peculiar as it is derived from both the internal and carotid artery systems (Figure 7.3). This confluent area provides the anatomical basis for any filler material that is inadvertantly injected into a nasal blood vessel to be propelled retrogradely into the orbit and thereby occlude the ophthalmic artery causing visual compromise.

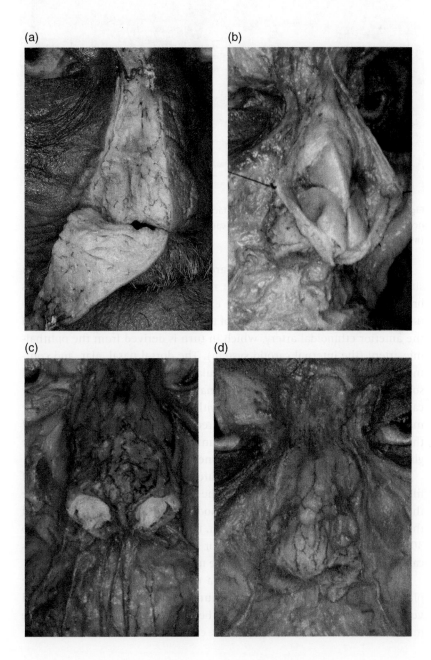

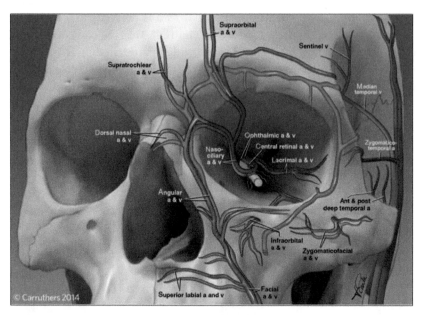

Figure 7.3 Vascular anatomy of the upper face showing the possible points of connection between the facial artery (external carotid system) and the ophthalmic artery (internal carotid system).

The columellar and alar arteries are the two main blood vessels that supply the lower two-thirds of the nose and are derived inferiorly as branches from the facial artery (the external carotid system). The dorsal nasal artery supplies the upper half of the nose and is a terminal branch of the anterior ethmoidal artery, which in turn is derived from the ophthalmic artery (the internal carotid system). The dorsal nasal, alar, and columellar arteries enter into a dense vascular plexus that covers the tip and soft tissue lobule of the nose. In some anatomical specimens the alar artery can be seen communicating directly with the dorsal nasal artery. All the major blood vessels of the nose are paired symmetrically on either side of the nose with a resultant watershed running down the midline from the glabellar down to the anterior nasal spine.

It would therefore appear that the safest way to deliver an injection of filler material to the nose is to stay on the midline and inject onto the bone therefore avoiding any of the major blood vessels that lie on the surface of the fibromuscular layer. For this reason, this author prefers to use a sharp 30G needle with a vertical approach for all injections on the nose as this can target the periosteal layer and bone most accurately.

Cannulae on the other hand have a tendency to glide in the middle plane of least resistance which unfortunately is where the major blood vessels lie. Larger bore cannulae may be intuitively safer but may cause more discomfort and the entry point can leave a visible mark on the nose. Furthermore, the cannula approach from the tip of the nose man-dates a parallel course to the dorsal arteries – a slightly off midline tra-jectory can result in the penetration of a relatively fixed dorsal artery. Once the cannula is within the vessel, it will remain there as it follows the pathway of least resistance, resulting in an intravascular event with disastrous consequences. This is evidenced by the fact that the author has received an anecdotal report from an experienced and senior col-league who recently injected a patient's nose using a large bore 21G cannula, inserted from the tip of the nose over the dorsum to the gla-bellar region, with retrograde injection. The surgeon noticed periorbital blanching almost immediately, after which the patient complained of blurred vision. Despite emergency cannulation of the supraorbital and supratrochlear arteries and infiltration of hyaluronidase, the patient became blind in one eye.

7.4 Indications

Injection rhinoplasty is indicated in patients who wish to have cosmetic enhancement of the nose without surgery. Younger patients are more concerned with correcting any percieved structural deficiencies and usu-ally request significant changes to the shapes of their noses. Older patients on the other hand are more appreciative of the rejuvenative effects that result from volumizing the root and bridge of the nose or uplifting a droop-ing tip. Ethnic considerations play a significant role in the choice of fillers.

Asian noses tend to be broad and flat with a low dorsum, a fleshy bul-bous tip, and widely spread alar lobules. Such noses require fillers with a high cohesivity to resist the contracting forces of the tight, thick overlying skin envelope to elevate the bridge, project the tip of the nose anteriorly, or to elongate the nose inferiorly. A small amount of filler placed lateral to the upper portion of the nasolabial fold can also displace the alar lobules medially, giving the impression of a narrower nasal base. (Figures 7.4a–d and 7.5a–d)

Caucasian noses usually have sufficient dorsal height and better pro-jection and definition of the tip due to the thinner skin envelope but may suffer from a dorsal hump, a narrow nasal bridge with an acute orbitonasal line, or a plunging tip. Fillers with a high cohesivity are desirable to provide structural support where it is needed, while fillers with a softer cohesivity can smoothen out the surface or contour irregularities better. A narrow nasal bridge with a 'pinched look' can easily be made more aesthetic by widening the root of the nose and tapering it towards the medial eyebrow (Figure 7.6a–d). Plunging tips can be elevated by providing support at the anterior nasal spine and the columella.

(a) (b)

(c) (d)

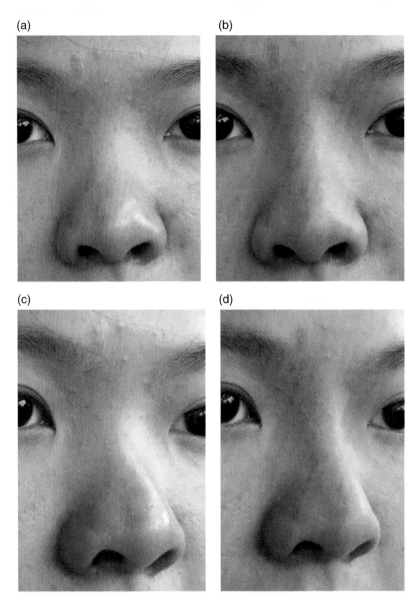

Figure 7.4 (a–d) A 22-year-old Asian woman requesting a higher nose bridge and more aesthetic naso-orbital line; 1.5 ml of hyaluronic acid filler was used to create significant elevation and 3-D contouring of the nasal bridge.

In the past, fillers were used only to augment the nasal dorsum but today, with a variety of fillers available that have different degrees of cohesivity, we can also achieve better sculpting and shaping of the tip, columella, and base of the nose. The aesthetic considerations for injection rhinoplasty should be no different to performing a surgical augmentation rhinoplasty, with the fillers taking the place of either the implant or any cartilage grafts.

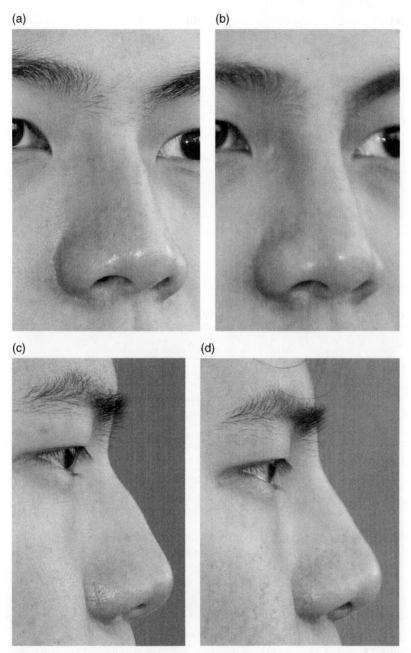

Figure 7.5 (a–d) A 28-year-old Asian man requesting a higher nasal bridge and tip projection. 2 cm³ of hyaluronic acid filler was used to achieve this result.

In some cases, such as blending the dorsal aesthetic line with the medial end of the brow (the orbitonasal line), a filler can be more useful than an implant alone as it creates an aesthetically smoother and curved transition between the side of the nose and the medial end of the eyebrow. Implants

(a)   (b)

(c)   (d)

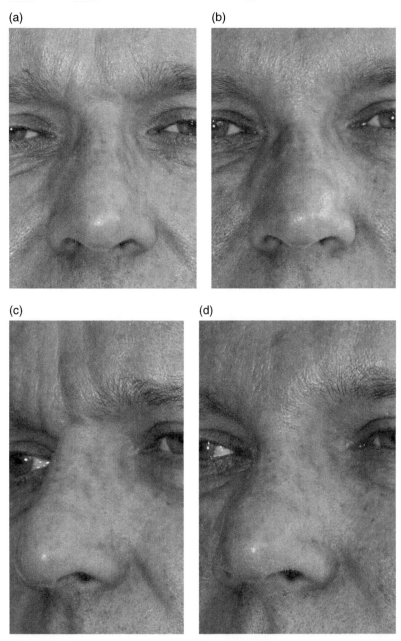

Figure 7.6 (a–d) A 49-year-old Caucasian man with deep glabellar and procerus frown lines, and an attenuated nasal root; 1 ml of hyaluronic acid filler was used to smoothen out the frown lines and to widen the root of the nose, providing aesthetic continuity with the medial brow: (a) frontal view pre-injection; (b) frontal view post-injection; (c) left oblique view pre-injection; (d) left oblique view post-injection.

on their own may actually aggravate the vertical glabellar furrows with a groove unaesthetically breaking up the continuous orbitonasal line [21].

7.5 Pain Relief

A useful trick prior to injecting the nose is to give a small amount (0.25 ml) of lidocaine 2% with adrenalin 1 : 200 000 to each of the supraorbital and infraorbital foramina, taking care not to allow the needle to enter into the foramina injuring either the blood vessels or the emerging nerves. This not only provides a degree of anaesthesia but also elicits a vasoconstriction of the blood vessels, which may reduce the risk of embolism. The local blocks are administered 10–15 minutes prior to the filler injections to allow adequate time for vasoconstriction to be achieved. Sometimes a blanching of the vascular territories can be seen. The use of an ice pack over the areas to be injected can also encourage vasoconstriction.

7.6 Injection Technique

Personal preference and the physician's own experience and familiarity with their tools will determine whether to use a cannula or a sharp needle to deliver the fillers to the nose. Equally good results can be obtained using either technique [22]. This author prefers the sharp needle technique using a half inch 30G needle for injecting the nose as it provides more 'feel' and aids in a more accurate placement of the fillers in the desired layer of the nose, which in most situations should be directly onto bone. Injection of the filler should always be preceded by aspiration to ensure a vessel has not been entered and the injection flow should be slow and steady. A 30G needle slows down the flow of injection and reduces rapid delivery under high pressure. Slowing down the injection also creates greater awareness of the volumization process and the subtle changes in nasal shape that can be achieved. As long as the injection is deep to the bone and in the midline, problems of vascular occlusion can be minimized. One must always be mindful of the underlying vascular anatomy and minimize the risks of vascular compromise.

7.6.1 The Six-Point Injection Technique for the Nose (Very Safe)

This is a simple, safe approach to augmenting the dorsum and tip of the nose as all the six injection points described are in the midline and injected deeply onto the bone or cartilage. A 30G needle is used and introduced perpendicularlly through the skin and soft tissue until the tip of the needle rests on the bone. The plunger is gently withdrawn to check for any backflow of blood. A bolus of filler is then slowly injected, keeping the pressure steady as the needle is withdrawn to the surface thereby creating a vertical column of filler, which having a broader base and a narrow apex (like a stalagmite) provides more structural support to tent up the overlying skin. By starting the injection on the bone, there is less likelihood of intravascular embolism and as the continuous vertical column of filler is created, any vessels in the path of the needle are displaced by the advancing edge of the filler. Each bolus delivered is no larger than 0.1–0.2 ml. Careful attention must be paid to any sudden blanching or intense pain felt by the patient that might indicate a vascular occlusion requiring immediate treatment with hyaluronidase.

Point 1 – this is the lowest point of the root of the nose usually at a level midway between the medial eyebrow and the medial canthus of the eye.

Point 2 – this is halfway between point 1 and the dorsal hump or K-point of the nose.

Point 3 – this point is just beyond the dorsal hump and will be injected onto the cartilaginous dorsum.

Point 4 – a point at the supratip depression

Point 5 – the entry point is at the apex of the tip of the nose and the needle is inserted perpendicularly down to the anterior nasal spine, traversing the columella between the medial crura. Here the injection starts deeply and as the needle is withdrawn linearly towards the tip, a horizontal structural beam of filler that projects the tip forward is created.

Point 6 – this point is slightly above point 5 and here the filler is injected intradermally or immmediately subdermal to shape the tip and create an aesthetic nuance (Figure 7.7a–f).

7.6.2 The Eight-Point Injection Technique for the Nose (Safe but may Have Risks)

This is the same as the six-point injection technique with the addition of two additional points (points 7 and 8) on either side of the midline and halfway between point 1 and the medial edge of the eyebrow (Figure 7.7g and h). This widens the root of the nose and creates a more aesthetic orbitonasal line. The injection should be deep onto the bone to avoid hitting a vessel. If the bolus is too large or the needle has strayed into the subcutaneous plane, vascular compromise with necrosis of the supratrochlear territory is a potential risk. An example of a patient receiving the eight-point injection technique is shown in (Figure 7.8a–f)

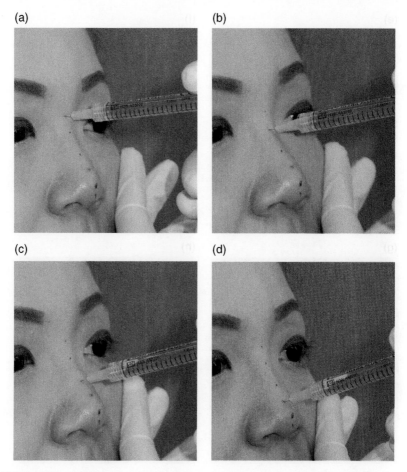

Figure 7.7 (a–h) Injection technique for nasal augmentation and contouring. The patient should be seated upright with the head resting comfortably on the back of the procedure chair. Supraorbital and infraorbital nerve blocks with 0.2 ml of lidocaine 2% with adrenaline 1 : 200 000 are administered for pain relief as well as intended vaso-constriction. Hyaluronic acid filler using a 30G needle is aimed perpendicularly down to the bone of the nasal radix in the midline. A small bolus is delivered directly onto the bone until the desired height of the nose is achieved. (b–d) The needle is removed and replaced at a point lower down from the previous injection to create a series of disconnected boluses that collectively create a slim aesthetic bridge. (e) A columellar strut is created by retrogradely injecting a long column of filler from the anterior nasal spine to the tip. This linear injection should pass deeply between the medial crura and not on its surface as the columellar arteries run superficially just under the skin of the columellar. (f) For additional tip projection and refinement a small amount of filler is injected intradermally or immediately subdermal in the midline of the tip thereby avoiding any major blood vessels. (g and h) Finally the nasal shape is completed by adding small boluses at either side of the radix to create a smoothly curved naso-orbital aesthetic line.

(e) (f)

(g) (h)

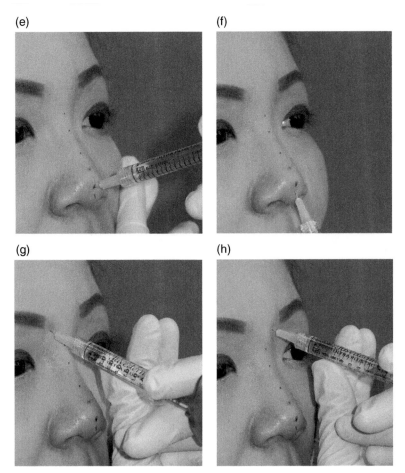

Figure 7.7 (Continued)

7.6.3 The Ten-Point Injection Technique for the Nose (Has More Risks)

This is not frequently performed. Two further points 9 and 10 are injected on either side of the alar lobule at the upper end of the nasolabial fold to narrow the apparent width of the nose. The filler is injected deeply as a bolus directly onto the bone by the side of the pyriform aperture, using slow steady pressure. These injections are more advanced and may potentially occlude a branch of or even the facial artery itself if improperly delivered. As long as the needle touches the bone, there is little risk of any vascular compromise as there are no major blood vessels on the periosteum. It is when the injection is given too super-ficially in this region that the risk increases as the facial artery is very superficial at this point.

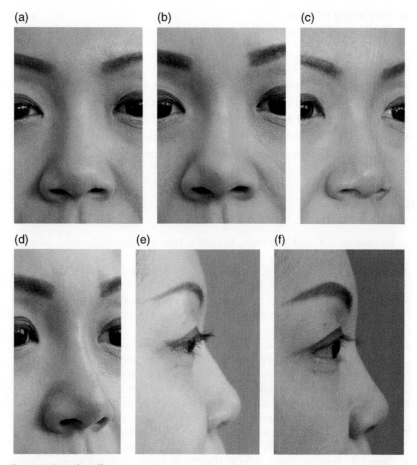

Figure 7.8 (a–f) Different pre-injection and post-injection views of a 40-year-old Asian woman wishing to have a higher nasal bridge, a smooth naso-orbital line, and better tip projection. The eight-point safe injection technique was used with 1.5 cm³ of hyaluronic acid filler.

7.7 Ten Tips for Good Injection Outcomes

1. Patients seated upright, head stable, good lighting.
2. You must be able to remove what you inject – therefore HA fillers are safest.
3. Use the least hydrophilic HA filler in your armamentarium.
4. Always have hyaluronidase mixed and ready before you start injecting. Severe complications can occur very quickly.
5. Use a 30G sharp needle for all injections as the needle tip can make direct contact with the bone or the cartilage; 30G needles slow down the injection speed and help you focus on delivering the correct amount of filler.

6. Stay in the midline.
7. Be aware of the underlying anatomical structures and stay away from bony foramina.
8. Be cautious of using a cannula as this tends to slip into the plane of least resistance, which is where the vessels are; it is difficult to keep the cannula tip in contact with the bone of the nasal dorsum.
9. Use lidocaine and adrenalin for local nerve blocks.
10. Avoid a long, continuous line of filler along the nasal bridge as this gives an unaesthetic sausage-like appearance.

References

1. De Lacerda, D.A. and Zancanaro, P. (2007). Filler rhinoplasty. *Dermatol. Surg.* 33: S207–S212.
2. Humphrey, C.D., Arkins, J.P., and Dayan, S.H. (2009 Nov–Dec). Soft tissue fillers in the nose. *Aesthet. Surg. J.* 29 (6): 477–484.
3. Piggot, J.R. and Yazdani, A. (2011 Winter). Hyaluronic acid used for the correction of nasal deviation in an 18 year old middle eastern man. *Can. J. Plast. Surg.* 19 (4): 156–158.
4. Redaelli, A. (2008). Medical rhinoplasty with hyaluronic acid and botulinum toxin A: a very simple and quite effective technique. *J. Cosmet. Dermatol.* 7: 210–220.
5. Liew, S., Wu, W.T.L., Chan, H.H. et al. (2015 Sep 25). Consensus on changing trends, attitudes, and concepts of Asian beauty. *Aesthet. Plast. Surg.* 40 (2): 193–201.
6. WTL, W., Liew, S., Chan, H.H. et al. (18 February 2016). Consensus on current injectable treatment strategies in the Asian face. *Aesthet. Plast. Surg.* 40 (2): 202–214.
7. Park, S.W., Woo, S.J., Park, K.H. et al. (Oct 2012). Iatrogenic retinal artery occlusion caused by cosmetic facial filler injections. *Am. J. Optom.* 154 (4): 653–662.
8. Lazzeri, S., Figus, M., Nardi, M. et al. (Feb 2013). Iatrogenic retinal artery occlusion caused by cosmetic facial filler injections. *Am. J. Optom.* 155 (2): 407–408.
9. Carruthers, J.D., Fagien, S., Rohrich, R.J. et al. (2014 Dec). Blindness caused by cosmetic filler injection: a review of cause and therapy. *Plast. Reconstr. Surg.* 134 (6): 1197–1201.
10. He, M.S., Sheu, M.M., Huang, Z.L. et al. (2013). Sudden bilateral vision loss and brain infarction following cosmetic hyaluronic acid injection. *JAMA Ophthalmol.* 131: 1234–1235.
11. Kim, E.G., Eom, T.K., and Kang, S.J. (2014). Severe visual loss and cerebral infarction after injection of hyaluronic acid gel. *J. Craniofac. Surg.* 25 (2): 684–686.
12. Kim, Y.J., Kim, S.S., Song, W.K. et al. (2011). Ocular ischemia with hypotony after injection of hyaluronic acid gel. *Ophthal. Plast. Reconstr. Surg.* 27 (6): 152–155.
13. Lazzeri, D., Agostini, T., Figus, M. et al. (2012 Apr). Blindness following cosmetic injections of the face. *Plast. Reconstr. Surg.* 129 (4): 995–1012.
14. Liu, O.G., Chunming, L., Juanjuan, W., and Xiaoyan, X. (2014). Central retinal artery occlusion and cerebral infraction following forehead injection with a corticosteroid suspension for vitiligo. *Indian J. Dermatol. Venereol. Leprol.* 80: 177–179.
15. Jiang, X., Liu, D.L., and Chen, B. (2014). Middle temporal vein: a fatal hazard in injection cosmetic surgery for temple augmentation. *JAMA Facial Plast. Surg.* 16 (3): 227–229.

16. Tansatit, T., Apinuntrum, P., and Phetudom, T. (Oct 2015). Temporal vein and the drainage vascular networks to assess the potential complications and the preventive maneuver during temporal augmentation using both anterograde and retrograde injections. *Aesthet. Plast. Surg.* 39 (5): 791–799.

17. De Lorenzi, C. (2014). Complications of injectable fillers, part 2: vascular complications. *Aesthet. Surg. J.* 34 (4): 584–600.

18. Beleznay, K., Carruthers, J.D.A., Humphrey, S., and Jones, D. (2015). Avoiding and treating blindness from fillers: a review of the world literature. *Dermatol. Surg.* 41 (10): 1097–1117.

19. Wu, W.T.L. (1992). The oriental nose: an anatomical basis for surgery. *Ann. Acad. Med. Singap.* 21: 176–189.

20. Saban, Y., Amodeo, C.A., Bouaziz, D., and Polselli, R. (2012). Nasal arterial vasculature: Medical and surgical applications. *Arch Facial Plast Surg.* 14 (6): 429–436.

21. Wu, W.T.L. (2009). Periorbital rejuvenation with injectable fillers. In: *Facial Rejuvenation with Fillers*, Techniques in Aesthetic Plastic Surgery Series (ed. S.R. Cohen and T.M. Born), 93–105. Saunders.

22. Wu, W., Carlisle, I., Huang, P. et al. (Feb 2010). Novel administration technique for large particle stabilised hyaluronic acid-based gel of non-animal origin in facial tissue augmentation. *Aesthet. Plast. Surg.* 34 (1): 88–95.

CHAPTER 8

The Lips

Shannon Humphrey

Carruthers & Humphrey Cosmetic Dermatology and University of British Columbia, Vancouver, British Columbia, Canada

8.1 Introduction

The lips can have a dramatic effect on overall appearance and play a critical role in sexual attraction, particularly in the flush of youth: slightly plump, with defined borders, a perfect Cupid's bow, and corners that curve gently upward. Since the introduction of collagen in the 1980s, the demand for lip augmentation has steadily grown. The introduction of longer-lasting but still impermanent soft-tissue fillers, such as hyaluronic acid (HA), has made a significant impact in the field of cosmetic dermatology, with 79% growth in the number of procedures over the past 6 years [1]. However, the augmented lip of early days – overfilled and duck-like in appearance – has given way to a more subtle effect, recreating the natural shape and contour of the lips as part of a global approach to restoring balance and harmony to the face as a whole.

8.2 In Search of Beautiful Proportions

Over the past thirty years, with the rising popularity of non-invasive techniques aimed at facial rejuvenation, much effort has been made to understand the qualities of a beautiful face. Research consistently identifies features considered attractive: a face that is oval in shape with large, round eyes, a small nose, and voluptuous lips [2]. Full lips impart a sense of youth, health, and sensuality [3]. Early Greek philosophers saw

---

Injectable Fillers: Facial Shaping and Contouring, Second Edition.
Edited by Derek H. Jones and Arthur Swift.
© 2019 John Wiley & Sons Ltd. Published 2019 by John Wiley & Sons Ltd.
Companion website: www.wiley.com/go/jones/injectable_fillers

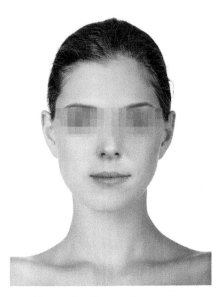

Figure 8.1 Ideal lip proportions and surface anatomy.

a strong connection between beauty and mathematics, describing it in terms of symmetry, harmony, and geometry [4]. In multiple studies of facial beauty, the single defining feature of beauty is symmetry, followed closely by balance and harmony [5]. One mathematical relationship has captured the interest of artists and scholars for thousands of years: the Golden Ratio or Divine Proportion, expressed as a mathematical ratio of 1 : 1.618, the number of Phi. The Golden Ratio has been reported to exist in all beautiful things, both living and innate, and this ratio can be seen in the beautiful lip [5]. In nature, the upper lip projects 2–3 mm more but is almost always smaller and less voluptuous than the lower lip. Within the Phi framework, the ideal vertical height ratio of upper to lower lip in youthful Caucasian lips is 1 : 1.6 [5, 6] (Figure 8.1). Exaggeration of these proportions or altering the ratio upsets the delicate balance between upper and lower lips [7].

8.2.1 Ethnic Variations

It goes without saying that lip morphology may differ amongst ethnic groups. Certainly, research has shown large, measurable differences between Asian, African, and Caucasian lips, particularly for lip fullness [8, 9]. Many African and Asian women genetically have a larger upper lip with a vertical height ratio of upper and lower lip that approaches 1 : 1. Many ethnic patients seek lip augmentation based on their cultural and racial background and do not aspire to the Western 'ideal'. It is critical to consider these ethnic variations and aesthetic preferences in the evaluation and treatment plan for lip augmentation to avoid inappropriate proportions and patient dissatisfaction [9].

8.3 The Ageing Lip

The perioral area is a significant aesthetic unit comprising the lip, oral commissures, nasolabial folds, and marionette lines. The upper lip is divided into three subunits, the well-known Cupid's bow, the central area of the upper lip vermilion, and vermilion-cutaneous junction (white roll). Philtral columns extend upward from each arc of the bow to the base of the columella on either side of the philtrum [10] (Figure 8.1).

Three factors contribute to age-related changes in the perioral region: dynamic muscular activity, volumetric changes due to bony resorption and fat pad reabsorption and redistribution, and intrinsic and extrinsic skin ageing.

Repetitive activity of the sphincteric orbicularis oris muscle causes the formation of fine perioral wrinkling around the lips, while the levator anguli oris, levator labii superioris alaeque nasi, zygomaticus major, and zygomaticus minor contribute to the formation of the nasolabial folds (Figure 8.2). Marionette lines are formed superiorly by cutaneous insertion of the depressor anguli oris (DAO) and inferiorly by the mandibular ligament [4].

During the ageing process, bony and soft tissue structures around the mouth and lips undergo significant alterations, resulting in changes to the shape and support of the lips [3]. The bony elements of the face provide the framework upon which soft tissues rest [11]. In the lower face, bone resorption causes maxillary retrusion and loss of mandibular height [11, 12]. Deep fat provides support for the overlying subcutaneous fat, which is partitioned into distinct anatomical departments [13]. Deflation, rather than descent, is the primary process in the ageing face, with significant atrophy of superficial and deep fat exacerbated by bony remodelling and subsequent contour changes [14, 15]. The effect of ageing in the

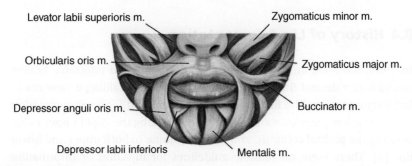

Figure 8.2 Perioral muscular anatomy.

face has been likened to a tablecloth draped over a table as it shrinks, causing the cloth to fold or sag [16].

Fat compartments in the perioral region are not as well characterized
as those in the upper face. Rohrich and Pessa defined multiple anatomical
compartments of subcutaneous fat that age independently [13]. Malar fat
is composed of three distinct medial, middle, and lateral temporal-cheek
fat compartments; the nasolabial fold is a discrete unit; and jowl fat represents the most inferior of the fat compartments. Cadaver research has
shown an area of fullness (the perioral mound) that lies at the junction
of the inferior most aspect of the malar superficial fat compartments and
the nasolabial folds [17]. Although it is unclear if the perioral mound is an
individual compartment or an extension or herniation of the nasolabial
compartment, it seems to be an area of fat deposition over time [17].

Ageing in the perioral region is a complex interplay of soft tissue changes
throughout the face; certainly, loss of volume and inferior descent of fat
from within the superficial and deep fat compartments in the upper face
contributes greatly to manifestations of ageing in the lower face, including the nasolabial folds, marionette lines, and jowls. Loss of volume in
subcutaneous fat deposits, ptosis of deep soft tissue, and laxity of ligaments causes the skin to droop, exacerbating lines and folds and drawing
attention to the lips. Nasolabial folds deepen, jowls emerge, and oral commissures turn downward, eventually forming into deeper marionette
lines [18]. Chronic activity of the orbicularis oris, combined with various
intrinsic and extrinsic factors, lead to dyspigmentation, irregular texture,
and the appearance of radial lip lines [7] (Figure 8.3).

The fundamental proportions of the lip – the Golden Ratio – change over
time. Volume is not necessarily lost but is redistributed along the length
of the lip [19], causing significant changes: the cutaneous portion of the
upper lip lengthens, while the upper lip vermilion thins. The lip margin
may become blunted, with a loss of definition to the philtral columns and
a flattening of the cupid's bow, while the lower lip thins and rolls inward
[4, 7, 18, 20].

8.4 History of Lip Augmentation

In 1981, the Food and Drug Administration approved injectable bovine
collagen as a dermal filler for the nasolabial fold, heralding a new era in
facial rejuvenation. The first reports of collagen used for lip augmentation
appeared a few years later and focused on enlarging the cupid's bow, exag-
gerating the philtral columns, and adding volume to both upper and lower
lips [3]. There were no sensible guidelines for injection or information
about proper aesthetic proportions. Lips were treated in isolation, and

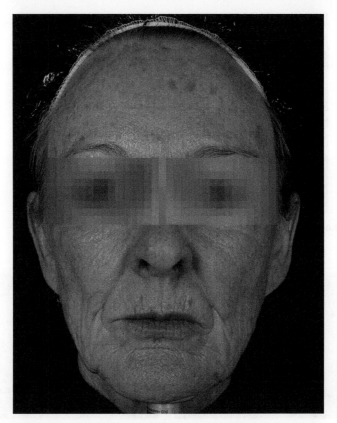

Figure 8.3 The perioral aesthetic unit and signs of skin ageing.

their treatment was readily apparent: the augmented lip of the 1980s was overinflated and out of proportion to the rest of the face (Figure 8.4).

Injectors eventually realized that the shape of the lips was as important as – if not more so than – volume, and that harmony in the face arises from proportion [21]. Today, lip augmentation is highly individualized, and the approach to treatment has widened to appreciate the lips in relationship to the face as a whole. Increased recognition of the effects of volume loss in the midface has meant a greater emphasis on providing support to the lower third of the face, not only by direct treatment of the lips themselves, but through volumetric restoration of the fat pads within the cheek, jaw, and chin. Because the ageing processes are intimately related and not seen in isolation, it is often necessary to rejuvenate the entire perioral complex [4]. Often, addressing fat loss and bony remodelling in the perioral region first, naturally results in a more beautiful lip, without any direct injection (Figure 8.5).

The modern lip is revitalized, rather than augmented, with subtle enhancement, proper proportioning of vertical height and length, and a

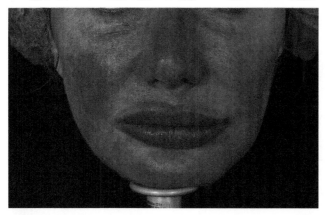

Figure 8.4 Historical overfilled 'duck lips'.

(a)   (b)

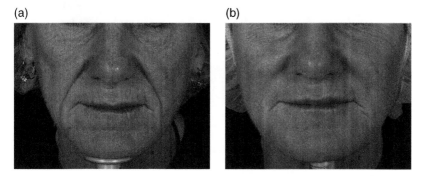

Figure 8.5 Improvement in the appearance of the lip before (a) and after (b) treatment of the supporting structures in the perioral region. (HA filler to deep cheek fat pads, prirform fossa, nasolabial folds, oral commissures and melomental folds) No treatment to vermillion lip.

distinct white roll. Lost surface structures have been redefined. The area around the mouth has been carefully treated to provide support and improve the natural shape of the lips in accordance with the patient's unique features, cultural background, and individual treatment goals.

8.5 Revitalization of the Lips

Because the lips and perioral anatomic subunit are so highly varied, it is nearly impossible to break down one treatment approach. There are many reasons for lip revitalization: to add volume globally, optimize the upper to lower lip ratio, widen the lip, add more definition, improve skin texture (Figure 8.6), further define the cupid's bow or philtral columns, to improve mouth corners, restore symmetry, soften radial lip rhytides,

(a)   (b)

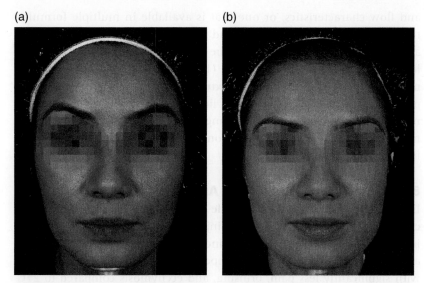

Figure 8.6 Textural improvement of vermillion lip before (a) and after (b) superficial injection of HA filler.

and any or all of the above. In every instance, treatment approach begins with a thorough anatomic assessment, not only of the lip itself, but also of the supporting structures around the lip. The shape and volume of the lip, the amount of vermilion show, the texture of the actual vermilion mucosa, and volume and support of the perioral region are all critical in the subsequent treatment plan and procedure.

8.5.1 Filler Options

The perioral region is unforgiving and sometimes difficult to treat, with the smallest mistake – either in placement of filler material or volume used – readily apparent. Repeated action of the orbicularis oris causes injected material to clump, leading to nodules, lumpiness, or product migration, especially with robust products of higher viscoelasticity [7]. Permanent agents or particulate fillers, such as polymethylmethacrylate and calcium hydroxylapatite, are associated with adverse effects such as nodules or delayed hypersensitivity reactions and are contraindicated for use in the lips. Although choice of filler material in the lips depends on several factors, including injector preference, area to be injected, and volume required, HA derivatives have become the treatment of choice for use in the delicate skin of the lips and in the perioral region due to ease of use and reversibility [22].

There are a number of HA formulations available. The optimal filler for placement in the lips and around the mouth is one that may be customized by blending with local anaesthetic or saline to adjust viscosity and flow characteristics, or one that is available in multiple formulations with various viscoelasticity and lift capabilities for use in different areas. The author prefers to use the Juvéderm® line of products (Allergan Inc., Irvine, CA): Volbella® (15 mg ml^{-1} HA) for soft enhancement in the body of the lip and a textural improvement with superficial placement; Volift® (17 mg ml^{-1}) for lip definition, mouth corners, and nasolabial folds; and Voluma® (20 mg ml^{-1}) for injection of the marionette lines. Voluma may also be reconstituted with 100% saline to treat fine perioral rhytides.

8.5.2 Needles, Cannulas, and Anaesthesia

Like choice of filler, the use of needle versus cannula depends on physician preference. Cannulae allow for injection of the entire lip using fewer injections, potentially reducing the incidence of local side effects. Fulton and colleagues found that blunt-tipped microcannulas were associated with significantly less pain, bruising, and ecchymosis compared to 27G needles when used for filler injections in the lips [23]. The author typically uses a 28G Excel needle or a 30G, 1.5″ cannula and BD 31G insulin syringe.

Lip injections can be painful. Historically, nerve blocks and lidocaine were used, but topical anaesthetic applied 30 minutes prior to injection combined with HA formulations premixed with lidocaine has made additional pain relief measures unnecessary. The application of ice packs before and after injections reduce swelling and tenderness.

8.5.3 Treatment Approach: Shape and Support

The approach to revitalization considers both the *shape* of the lips, as well as the *support* provided to the lower third of the face [3]. In the ageing individual with considerable volume loss in the lower face, increasing the amount of support in the tissues around the mouth – in the midface, along the nasolabial folds and marionette lines, and in the jaw – is more important than injecting the lips directly.

The art of beautifying the lips themselves revolves around subtle enhancement and restoration of definition, symmetry, and balance, with two basic goals: recreation or redefinition of a distinct upper lip white roll, followed by proper proportioning of vertical height and lip length [5]. Older patients often require redefinition of the structural landmarks of the lip. A video of the author injecting a lip accompanies this chapter. Treating the vermilion border first provides the framework for subsequent revolumization and may improve fine perioral wrinkling [20]. The author typically begins in the lateral upper lip and moves medially, depositing filler along the white line to the philtral column base (see videos). Injection of filler along the philtral columns using a threading technique improves the contours of the lip and the Cupid's bow, while subsequent injections into the wet roll on either side of the columns add fullness and shape [18, 20]. Recognizing the areas of natural prominence – one in the midline of the upper lip, one laterally on each side of the upper lip, and one just lateral to the midline on each side of the lower lip – helps to identify injection sites [7]. In the lower lip, injections into the wet roll elevate the corners of the mouth and may reduce the depth of the marionette lines.

8.6 Combination Therapy

The perioral region is particularly susceptible to all factors of intrinsic and extrinsic ageing, with associated changes to skin colour, tone, and texture. In most patients – including those with pronounced radial lip lines, for example, or severe photodamage – optimal revitalization of the perioral region involves a comprehensive treatment regimen combining two or more modalities, particularly botulinum toxin type A (BoNT-A) and energy-based treatments for tightening and improvements in texture (Figure 8.7).

8.6.1 Botulinum Toxin

The benefits of combination therapy using fillers and BoNT-A have been well documented [24–26]. BoNT-A minimizes muscle contraction, extending the duration of the filler implant, and is particularly useful for perioral rejuvenation [26]. In a systematic comparison of BoNT-A and HA alone

(a)   (b)

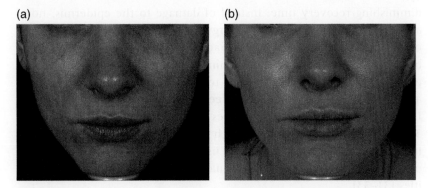

Figure 8.7 Patient before (a) and after (b) combination therapy using poly-l-lactic acid to piriform fossa, 4u Onabotulinum toxin A to perioral region, photorejuvenation, non-ablative fractionated laser (1440mn) and radiofrequency to lower face.

or in combination to treat the ageing lower face, combination therapy provided greater degrees of overall improvement in addition to longer-lasting effects [26]. Small doses of BoNT-A around the lips may improve the appearance of radial lip lines [4]. The author prefers to use a 2.5 ml dilution for her onabotulinumtoxinA 100 U using a dose range between 3 and 8 U. In younger individuals, minor downturn of the oral commissures – caused by the strength of the platysma and DAO muscles – may be corrected easily with BoNT-A; injection into the DAO relieves the depressor action on the oral commissures and allows the levator muscles to act without opposition, lifting the mouth corners while enhancing the longevity of the filling agent [20]. Constant mobility in the perioral region tends to decrease the longevity of BoNT-A; touch-ups are typically required every two to three months.

8.6.2 Resurfacing and Energy-based Therapies

A comprehensive rejuvenation approach often includes some form of ablative resurfacing or non-ablative remodelling to fully restore vitality [4]. Ablative procedures damage the epidermis and dermis, initiating the tissue-repair cascade, in which inflammatory mediators induce fibroblasts to generate new collagen and elastin, ultimately leading to remodelling of the skin with dramatic improvements. Microdermabrasion, chemical peels, and carbon dioxide (CO_2) or erbium: yttrium aluminium garnet (Er:YAG) lasers provide various degrees of resurfacing. Ablative lasers, in particular, produce unparalleled results but are associated with a significant period of recovery and adverse events, including the risk of scarring [27, 28].

As a result, ablative technology has largely been replaced by non-ablative modalities that induce dermal neocollagenesis with minimal epidermal disruption, reducing the risk of adverse events and diminishing recovery time. Instead of damage to the epidermis, non-ablative devices direct thermal energy to the reticular dermis and subcutis, where immediate tissue contraction and delayed remodelling are believed to cause collective tightening and lifting of the skin. Intense pulsed light (IPL) has been shown to improve skin texture, pore size, and fine lines; in individuals with deeper, dynamic rhytides, combining IPL with concomitant BoNT provides better results than IPL alone [29, 30]. Skin tightening treatments with radiofrequency devices and high-intensity focused ultrasound can be used to soften fine lines in the perioral region and work well in combination with BoNT and other modalities [31–33].

8.7 Side Effects and Complications

Common injection-related side effects include pain, bruising, and swelling that are typically mild and resolve within a few days [9]. The lips are particularly prone to hematoma and injury [34].Significant swelling typically settles within one to two days; however, subtle swelling can persist for up to 10–14 days. It is preferable not to adjust any treatment until all of the swelling has resolved to allow for an accurate clinical assessment.

Complications in the lips are rare but include irregularities, asymmetries, and palpable areas, which often may be attributed to inappropriate choice of filler or injection techniques [18]. The perioral region is largely unforgiving, and a conservative approach with small-volume injections is recommended, allowing for subsequent touch-ups one to two weeks after the initial treatments, if necessary. This approach will reduce the severity of injection-related side effects and avoid overcorrection. Too much product placed too superficially may lead to clumping, beading, and visibility of the implant (Figure 8.8). Nodule formation and hypersensitivity reactions are largely associated with permanent or particulate fillers but have also been reported after treatment with HA [35].

A thorough understanding of the placement of perioral vasculature is critical. Vent and colleagues investigated nine women treated for augmentation of the lips and perioral region with HA and found that while no serious complications occurred, injections came perilously close to important structures, such as blood vessels [36]. Branches of the facial

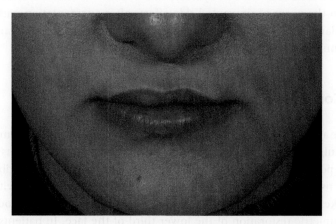

Figure 8.8 Side effect of superficial placement of HA filler showing nodularity.

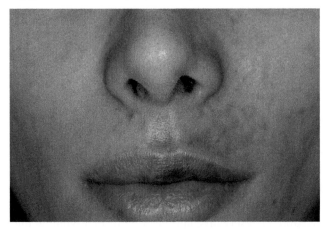

Figure 8.9 Vascular occlusion 1.5 days after HA filler to lips. Source: Figure courtesy of David Zloty MD FRCPC.

artery – the inferior and superior labial arteries – run along the edges of the upper and lower lips. Vascular occlusion is a rare but potentially serious complication that may occur after inadvertent injection of filler into the labial artery, resulting in vascular compromise, occlusion, or tissue necrosis [37] (Figure 8.9). Treatment measures include injection of hyaluronidase, warm compresses, massage and, for certain patients, administration of aspirin, prednisone, and typical nitroglycerin paste at the first sign of compromise and impending necrosis.

Hyaluronidase – a soluble protein enzyme that acts at the site of local injection to break down and hydrolyse HA – is an essential tool to keep on hand in the event of unwanted side effects after augmentation with HA, particularly for use in the lip, as even the subtlest over-correction can look very unnatural [38].

8.8 Conclusion

Lips are a dramatic and defining feature of an attractive face. Over time, the beautiful, defined arched structure of the upper lip is lost, and in its place a thin, poorly defined upper lip develops, with atrophy and redistribution of soft tissue leading to significant alterations [4]. Modern lip revitalization takes into account the role of ageing on the face as a whole, focusing on volumetric restoration of the lower third of the face. In patients with significant ageing and volume loss in the perioral region, renewing support through volume augmentation in the supporting structures around the mouth is more important than filling the lip itself and often improves fine lines and natural lip proportions. Tailoring treatment to individual anatomy, ethnic background, and personal goals will optimize outcomes. In individuals with severe ageing, volume loss, and signs of photodamage, a comprehensive approach combining multiple rejuvenation modalities may be required.

References

1. American Society for Dermatologic Surgery. (2017). 2017 dermatologic proce-dures data. Retrieved October 1, 2018 from https://www.asds.net/portals/0/PDF/procedure-survey-results-infographic-2017.pdf
2. Etcoff, N. (1999). *Survival of the Prettiest: The Science of Beauty*. New York: Doubleday.
3. Klein, A.W. (2005). In search of the perfect lip: 2005. *Dermatol. Surg.* 31 (11 Pt 2): 1599–1603.
4. Perkins, N.W., Smith, S.P. Jr., and Williams, E.F. 3rd. (2007). Perioral rejuvenation: complementary techniques and procedures. *Facial Plast. Surg. Clin. North Am.* 15: 423–432.
5. Swift, A. and Remington, K. (2011). BeautiPHIcation: a global approach to facial beauty. *Clin. Plast. Surg.* 28: 347–377.
6. Mandy, S. (2007). Art of the lip. *Dermatol. Surg.* 33: 521–522.
7. Sarnoff, D.S. and Gotkin, R.H. (2012). Six steps to the "perfect" lip. *J. Drugs Dermatol.* 11: 1081–1088.
8. Wong, W.W., Davis, D.G., Camp, M.C., and Gupta, S.C. (2010). Contribution of lip proportions to facial aesthetics in different ethnicities: a three-dimensional analysis. *J. Plast. Reconstr. Aesthet. Surg.* 63: 2032–2039.
9. Nelson, A.A., Callendar, V.D., Kim, J., and Beddingfield, F.C. (2013). Lip augmenta-tion. In: *Procedures in Cosmetic Dermatology: Soft-Tissue Augmentation* (ed. J. Carruthers and A. Carruthers), 140–146. London: Elsevier Saunders.
10. Maloney, B.P., Truswell, W. 4th, and Waldman, S.R. (2012). Lip augmentation: discussion and debate. *Facial Plast. Surg. Clin. North Am.* 20: 327–346.
11. Shaw, R.B. Jr., Katzel, E.B., Koltz, P.F. et al. (2010). Aging of the mandible and its aesthetic implications. *Plast. Reconstr. Surg.* 125: 332–342.
12. Pessa, J.E., Slice, D.E., Hanz, K.R. et al. (2008). Aging and the shape of the mandible. *Plast. Reconstr. Surg.* 121: 196–200.
13. Rohrich, R.J. and Pessa, J.E. (2007). The fat compartments of the face: anatomy and clinical implications for cosmetic surgery. *Plast. Reconstr. Surg.* 119: 2219–2227.
14. Lambros, V. (2008). Models of facial aging and implications for treatment. *Clin. Plast. Surg.* 35: 319–327.
15. Fitzgerald, R., Graivier, M.H., Kane, M. et al. (2010). Update on facial aging. *Aesthet. Surg. J.* 30 (Suppl): 11S–24S.
16. Vleggaar, D. and Fitzgerald, R. (2008). Dermatological implications of skeletal aging: a focus on supraperiosteal volumization for perioral rejuvenation. *J. Drugs Dermatol.* 7: 209–220.

17. Sullivan, P.K., Hoy, E.A., Mehan, V., and Singer, D.P. (2010). An anatomical evaluation and surgical approach to the perioral mound in facial rejuvenation. *Plast. Reconstr. Surg.* 126: 1333–1340.

18. Sclafani, A.P. (2005). Soft tissue fillers for management of the aging perioral complex. *Facial Plast. Surg.* 21: 74–78.

19. Iblher, N., Kloepper, J., Penna, V. et al. (2008). Changes in the aging upper lip – a photomorphometric and MRI-based study (on a quest to find the right rejuvenation approach). *J. Plast. Reconstr. Aesthet. Surg.* 61: 1170–1176.

20. Wollina, U. (2013). Perioral rejuvenation: restoration of attractiveness in aging females by minimally invasive procedures. *Clin. Interv. Aging* 8: 1149–1155.

21. Tessier, P. (1987). Foreward. In: *Anthropometric Facial Proportions in Medicine* (ed. L.G. Farkas and I.R. Munro), ix–x. Springfield: Charles C. Thomas.

22. Carruthers, J.D., Glogau, R.G., and Blitzer, A. (2008). Facial aesthetics consensus group faculty. Advances in facial rejuvenation: botulinum toxin type a, hyaluronic acid dermal fillers, and combination therapies – consensus recommendations. *Plast. Reconstr. Surg.* 121 (5 Suppl): 5S–30S.

23. Fulton, J., Caperton, C., Weinkle, S., and Dewandre, L. (2012). Filler injections with the blunt-tip microcannula. *J. Drugs Dermatol.* 11: 1098–1103.

24. Carruthers, J. and Carruthers, A. (2003). A prospective, randomized, parallel group study analyzing the effect of BTX-A (Botox) and nonanimal sourced hyaluronic acid (NASHA, Restylane) in combination compared with NASHA (Restylane) alone in severe glabellar rhytides in adult female subjects: treatment of severe glabellar rhytides with a hyaluronic acid derivative compared with the derivative and BTX-A. *Dermatol. Surg.* 29: 802–809.

25. Coleman, K.R. and Carruthers, J. (2006). Combination therapy with BOTOX and fillers: the new rejuvenation paradigm. *Dermatol. Ther.* 19: 177–188.

26. Carruthers, A., Carruthers, J., Monheit, G.D. et al. (2010). Multicenter, randomized, parallel-group study of the safety and effectiveness of onabotulinumtoxinA and hyaluronic acid dermal fillers (24-mg/ml smooth, cohesive gel) alone and in combination for lower facial rejuvenation. *Dermatol. Surg.* 36 (Suppl 4): 2121–2134.

27. Janik, J.P., Markus, J.L., Al-Dujaili, Z., and Markus, R.F. (2007). Laser resurfacing. *Semin. Plast. Surg.* 21: 139–146.

28. Alam, M. and Warycha, M. (2011). Complications of lasers and light treatments. *Dermatol. Ther.* 24: 571–580.

29. Khoury, J.G., Saluja, R., and Goldman, M.P. (2008). The effect of botulinum toxin type a on full-face intense pulsed light treatment: a randomized, double-blind, split-face study. *Dermatol. Surg.* 34: 1062–1069.

30. Goldberg, D.J. (2012). Current trends in intense pulsed light. *J. Clin. Aesthet. Dermatol.* 5: 45–53.

31. Lolis, M.S. and Goldberg, D.J. (2012). Radiofrequency in cosmetic dermatology: a review. *Dermatol. Surg.* 38: 1765–1776.

32. MacGregor, J.L. and Tanzi, E.L. (2013). Microfocused ultrasound for skin tightening. *Semin. Cutan. Med. Surg.* 32: 18–25.

33. Minkis, K. and Alam, M. (2014). Ultrasound skin tightening. *Dermatol. Clin.* 32: 71–77.

34. Pinar, Y.A., Bilge, O., and Govsa, F. (2005). Anatomic study of the blood supply of perioral region. *Clin. Anat.* 18: 330–339.

35. Ledon, J.A., Savas, J.A., Yang, S. et al. (2013). Inflammatory nodules following soft tissue filler use: a review of causative agents, pathology and treatment options. *Am. J. Clin. Dermatol.* 14: 401–411.

36. Vent, J., Lefarth, F., Massing, T., and Angerstein, W. (2014). Do you know where your fillers go? An ultrastructural investigation of the lips. *Clin. Cosmet. Investig. Dermatol.* 7: 191–199.

37. Beleznay, K., Humphrey, S., Carruthers, J., and Carruthers, A. (2014 Sep). Vascular compromise from soft tissue augmentation: experience with 12 cases and recommendations for optimal outcomes. *J. Clin. Aesthet. Dermatol.* 7: 37–43.

38. Humphrey, S. and Weiss, R.A. (2013). Reversers. In: *Procedures in Cosmetic Dermatology: Soft-Tissue Augmentation* (ed. J. Carruthers and A. Carruthers), 200–207. London: Elsevier Saunders.

CHAPTER 9

The Mandible, Jawline, and Chin

Amir Moradi and Jeff Watson

Moradi M.D., Vista, CA, USA

9.1 Introduction

The ageing face undergoes what appears to be a redistribution of volume from the upper to the lower face as changes occur within the soft tissue and bony architecture. Resorption and atrophy of the malar, submalar, and buccal fat pockets leads to volume loss in the midface. Concurrently, the lower third of the face widens and the face transitions from the heart-shaped frame that is a hallmark of youth to a more square appearance that is less aesthetically appealing. Pivotal in this process are changes along the jawline, which even when subtle, begin to signify advancing age.

Loss of jawline definition is multifactorial. Increased skin laxity, incongruent changes in subcutaneous tissue and mandibular bone resorption lead to the loss of definition of a straight mandibular line, the formation of jowls, and a deepening of the pre-jowl sulcus. The labiomandibular folds, which are fixed by the mandibular ligament, become increasingly prominent and further draw attention to the region. These shifts in volume and position of the soft tissue of the lower face result in age-specific shadowing patterns that detract from a patient's appearance. The use of synthetic fillers allows one to adjust the soft tissue contour along the mandible to improve or eliminate undesirable shadows and to restore youthful definition to the jawline.

Injectable rejuvenation focuses on two key areas, the angle of the mandible and the jowl/pre-jowl region. Augmentation of the pre-jowl sulcus camouflages the soft tissue descent of the jowl and re-establishes the

Injectable Fillers: Facial Shaping and Contouring, Second Edition.
Edited by Derek H. Jones and Arthur Swift.
© 2019 John Wiley & Sons Ltd. Published 2019 by John Wiley & Sons Ltd.
Companion website: www.wiley.com/go/jones/injectable_fillers

contour of inferior mandibular border. At the angle of the mandible, individuals who have always had a poorly defined jawline or those who have lost volume with age, benefit significantly from improved definition here. The combined approach addressing the pre-jowl region and mandibular angle results in a natural and smooth transition along the jawline from mentum to angle that is both youthful and attractive.

9.2 Regional Anatomy

At the angle of the mandible the key tissue layers from superficial to deep include the skin, subcutaneous fat, superficial musculoaponeurotic system (SMAS), masseteric fascia, masseter, periosteum, and mandibular cortex. The masseter originates along the inferior border of the zygomatic arch and inserts at the angle of the mandible and the ascending mandibular ramus. The so-called masseteric ligaments arise from the anterior border of the masseter and insert into the SMAS and overlying skin. Age-related relaxation of these ligaments contributes to the formation of jowls. The posterior portion of the masseter along the ramus of the mandible is covered by the parotid gland. The parotid duct traverses the lateral surface of the masseter before wrapping around the anterior border, where it pierces the buccinator and ultimately enters the oral cavity.

In the pre-jowl region, the key soft tissue layers include the skin, the superficial fat compartment, the platysma fusing into the depressor anguli oris (DAO), the deep fat compartment, and bone. More anteriorly, the DAO obliquely overlaps the depressor labii inferioris (DLI) along the inferior border of the mandibular parasymphysis.

The principle vessels of concern to the injector are the facial artery and vein. The facial artery arises from the external carotid artery and travels deep to the platysma crossing over the body of the mandible approximately 3–3.5 cm anterior to the mandibular angle before heading anteriorly towards the oral commissure (Figures 9.1 and 9.2). One can frequently palpate the location of the facial artery by its pulsation or by feeling for the depression of the antegonial notch where the facial artery crosses the inferior border of the mandible, just anterior to the border of the masseter muscle. The facial vein descends just posterior to the facial artery, crossing the inferior border of the mandible approximately 2.5 cm anterior medially, passing through the orbicularis oris and the lip depressors. Multiple small branches to the angle continuing inferiorly into the neck (Figures 9.1 and 9.2).

The facial artery takes a tortuous course as it heads towards the corner of the mouth. The inferior labial artery (ILA) arises from the labiomental branch of the facial artery and travels perpendicularly from the ILA towards

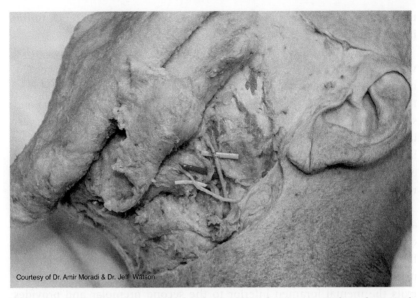

Courtesy of Dr. Amir Moradi & Dr. Jeff Watson

Figure 9.1 Cadaver dissection of the facial vein (blue), facial artery (red), and marginal mandibular branch of the facial nerve (yellow).

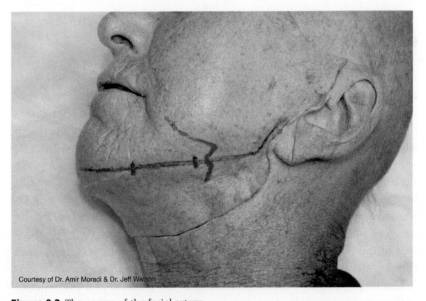

Courtesy of Dr. Amir Moradi & Dr. Jeff Watson

Figure 9.2 The course of the facial artery.

the lower lip where it joins in an anastomotic arcade [1]. The main trunk of the facial artery continues superiorly, passing approximately 1.5 cm lateral to the oral commissure and then branches to form the superior labial artery (SLA) which travels medially along the upper lip [2]. The vascular supply to the chin consists of an anastomotic network fed by branches of the labiomental artery, inferior labial artery, and the mental branch of the inferior alveolar artery.

Motor innervation to the mimetic muscles of the lower face is carried via the buccal and marginal mandibular branches of the facial nerve. The marginal mandibular nerve exits the substance of the parotid gland posterior to the angle of the mandible then courses deep to the platysma and superficial to the facial artery and vein. Anatomic studies demonstrate variability in the path along the jawline, where it may run either above or below the border of the mandible until it crosses over the facial artery and at that point predictably heads superiorly and anteriorly towards the corner of the mouth [3].

Sensory innervation in the region is supplied by the both the trigeminal and cervical nerves. At the angle of the mandible, sensory innervation is carried by the great auricular nerve (C2, C3). The skin over the lateral surface of the body of the mandible is innervated by the buccal branch of the mandibular nerve (V3) that extends to the jowls. The mental nerve (V3) exits the mental foramen inferior to the second premolar and provides sensation to the pre-jowl area and chin. One must approach this region gingerly as it can be very sensitive for patients.

9.3 Aesthetic Ideals

Achieving the ideal aesthetic outcome in augmenting the jawline rests upon proper assessment of the patient's bony structure, soft tissue, and skin quality as they pertain to age-related changes in the region. Understanding the aesthetic ideals as well as key differences in men and in women will allow the injector to form a treatment plan with a clearly defined goal.

Examination of the patient is performed with the patient in an upright sitting position, with the head positioned in Frankfort plane. The soft tissue in this region is mobile and thus changes significantly depending on head and neck position. The injector must have room to move around the treatment chair to evaluate the patient from all angles including visualization of the inferior border of the mandible. Pretreatment photographs of frontal, lateral and oblique views should be taken at a minimum.

Assessment begins with an evaluation of the position and prominence of the mandibular angle. A youthful jawline is well-defined with a smooth uninterrupted trajectory from the mentum to the angle of the mandible. The ideal position for the mandibular angle lies at the intersection of the inferior border of the mandible with a line drawn parallel to the angle of the auricle and positioned just in front of the tragus. On cephalometric evaluation, this angle is ideally 128° [4]. This may be visualized by the injector or marked on the skin as a topographic guide prior to injection.

The thickness of the skin and subcutaneous tissue overlying the mandible must be appreciated as it will serve as a guide to choosing the appropriate product. Asymmetries should be appreciated and brought to the attention of the patient prior to the procedure. Lastly, a history of facial procedures and surgeries must be obtained and any sequelae noted.

9.4 Treatment Modality and Product Choice

There are a variety of treatment modalities, both non-surgical and surgical, that have been used to address the jawline, each with varying degrees of invasiveness and risk. Traditionally, the jawline has been addressed by a facelift procedure in which patients can expect a significant reduction of the jowls and marked improvement of jawline definition. Fat augmentation [5] has also been used in the jawline as have sutures [6] with varying degrees of efficacy. The expanding filler market and increasing patient demand has demonstrated that a significant proportion of patients are interested in less invasive rejuvenation with decreased risk and recovery time, but with immediately visible results.

The treatment modalities for chin augmentation include genioplasty, synthetic chin implants, and injectable fillers. To determine the ideal chin projection, we use the relationship between the vermilion border of the lower lip to the gnathion as a guide [7]. Although we keep the entire facial structure under consideration, we have found this relationship to be very useful. Ideally, the gnathion needs to be within 5 mm of a vertical tangential line to the vermillion border of the lower lip, when the head is positioned in the Frankfort horizontal plan and evaluated from a lateral position. As a general rule, we use the distance between the oral commissure and vermillion boarder as a general guide when evaluating the chin projection.

The available products best suited for jawline augmentation include solid particles of calcium hydroxylapatite (Radiesse®, Merz) and a highly elastic hyaluronic acid such as Juvederm® Voluma® XC (Allergan), or Restylane® Lyft (Galderma).

An examination of the patient to determine the respective bony and soft tissue structure along the jawline serves to guide the injector to the best product or combination of products to use. A patient with thin skin over a well-defined and prominent mandible requires soft tissue augmentation and is best served with use of a compressible filler such as Juvederm Voluma XC or Restylane Lyft. When the skin and soft tissue layers are thicker and the bony structure of the mandible is poorly defined, the patient requires rigid structural augmentation with an incompressible filler, such as Radiesse, to improve definition of the bony structure and to support the overlying tissues. In a patient with thick skin, soft tissue, and a reasonably well-defined mandibular structure, either product or a mixture of Radiesse with a hyaluronic acid in varying concentrations can be used. Commonly, either category of filler can be used with good result, but in the cases listed earlier, the proper choice of either Juvederm Voluma XC, Restylane Lyft, or Radiesse will provide the ideal aesthetic outcome. One should remember that only hyaluronic acids are reversible with hyaluronidase.

9.5 Injection Technique

9.5.1 Mandible and Jaw Line
Topical or local anaesthetic can be used for patient comfort. The skin needs to be prepped with the proper antiseptic solution to decrease the risk of infection. It may be helpful to mark the optimal aesthetic location of the mandibular angle on the skin. The injections need to be placed in the subcutaneous tissue between the bone and subdermal layer. When using the cannula technique the tip of the cannula is continuously and slowly moved while small aliquots of less than 0.1 cm³ are placed between the periosteum and subcutaneous tissue. When using the needle technique multiple entries are performed through the skin and similarly small aliquots of less than 0.1 cm³ are placed between the periosteum and subcutaneous tissue. It is best to keep the injection volumes between 0.01 and 0.1 cm³ per insertion, and massage frequently. The injection technique is demonstrated in the accompanied live patient injection video (Video 9.1) with representative before and after images (Figures 9.3 and 9.4). While the authors demonstrate augmentation using a needle in the video that accompanies this chapter, a cannula may also be used, which may provide additional safety against vascular injury.

9.5.2 Chin Augmentation
The injection plan is in the deep subcutaneous tissue, as close to the bone as possible. Both the projection and the height of the chin can be enhanced by placement of the filler anterior and inferior to the mandibular symphysis. The injection volumes should be limited to less than 0.02–0.1 cm³ per injection and massaged frequently.

9.6 Post-procedure Care

The patient is counselled regarding swelling, bruising, and pain with mastication. Patients are discharged with a cold compress. Twice daily massage for two to three minutes is recommended for three days after the procedure.

(a)   (b)

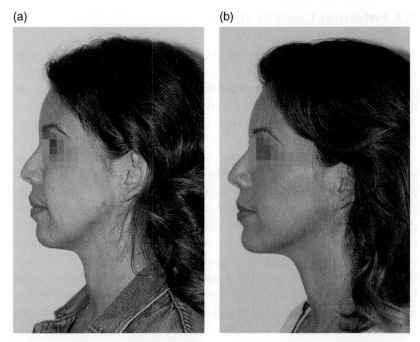

Figure 9.3 Jawline rejuvenation with calcium hydroxylapatite before (a) and after (b) treatment.

(a)   (b)

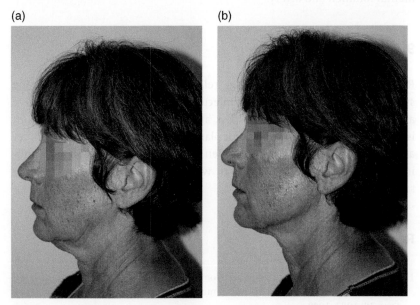

Figure 9.4 Jawline rejuvenation with calcium hydroxylapatite before (a) and after (b) treatment.

9.7 Potential Complications

When performed according to the technique described earlier and with an understanding of the relevant regional anatomy, filler administration along the jawline is very safe. Most adverse events include swelling and bruising, which usually resolve in 7–10 days. Other complications that may arise include asymmetry, irregularities, or infection. The authors recommend small volumes of 0.1 ml or less per injection point both for safety reasons and for better aesthetic outcome. Although pulling back on the syringe prior to injection is frequently discussed as a safety precaution to prevent the devastating sequelae of intravascular injection, the authors suggest that this is not always reliable and may lead to a false sense of security. Administration of the filler outside the course of the facial artery and vein, combined with small bolus injection technique, represent the most consistently safe approach to the region. Inadvertent injection of filler into the inferior labial artery may lead to vascular compromise of the ipsilateral lower lip and can be avoided by deep injection along the bone. The chin may theoretically be at lower risk of vascular compromise given its rich anastomotic network from multiple feeding arteries; however, deep injection on bone is nonetheless recommended to avoid any potential complications. Care should be taken not to inject on bone in the area of the mental foramen and artery.

9.8 Conclusion

Refined techniques to address age-related changes to the jawline using synthetic fillers has allowed the injector to restore a youthful, attractive appearance to patients with low risk and minimal downtime. Paramount is proper assessment and treatment planning that guide the choice of filler and location of administration. When performed properly, an outstanding aesthetic result can be achieved with both high patient and injector satisfaction.

References

1. Tansatit, T., Apinuntrum, P., and Phetudom, T. (2014). A typical pattern of the labial arteries with implication for lip augmentation with injectable fillers. *Aesthet. Plast. Surg.* 38: 1083–1089.
2. Pinar, Y.A., Bilge, O., and Govsa, F. (2005). Anatomic study of the blood supply of perioral region. *Clin. Anat.* 18: 330–339.

3. Potgieter, W., Meiring, J., Boon, J. et al. (2005 Apr). Mandibular landmarks as an aid in minimizing injury to the marginal mandibular branch: a metric and geometric anatomical study. *Clin. Anat.* 18 (3): 171–178.
4. Rakowski, T. (1982). *An Atlas and Manual of Cephalometry Radiography*. Philadelphia: Lea & Febiger.
5. Coleman, S.R. (2006). Facial augmentation with structural fat grafting. *Clin. Plast. Surg.* 33 (4): 567–577.
6. Abraham, R.F., DeFatta, R.J., and Williams, E.F. (2009). Thread-lift for facial rejuvenation: assessment of long-term results. *Arch. Facial Plast. Surg.* 11 (3): 178–183.
7. Simons, R.L. (1975). Adjunctive measures in rhinoplasty. *Otolaryngol. Clin. N. Am.* 8: 717–742.

CHAPTER 10

Submental Contouring

Frederick C. Beddingfield III[1], Jeanette M. Black[2],
Paul F. Lizzul[1], and Ardalan Minokadeh[2]

[1] Sienna Biopharmaceuticals, Westlake Village, CA, USA

[2] Skin Care and Laser Physicians of Beverly Hills, Los Angeles, CA, USA

The appearance of the neck and chin have a substantial impact on overall facial aesthetics and self-perception. An elegant neck contour contributes to overall facial balance, and in men, a strong chin is generally associated with authority, self-confidence, and trustworthiness [1]. For a youthful and aesthetic neck, the cervicomental angle should ideally measure between 105 and 120°; an angle greater than 120°, commonly caused by excess submental fat (SMF), can lead to an undesirable appearance of submental convexity/fullness (double chin) [2]. In a consumer survey conducted by the American Society for Dermatologic Survey in 2015, 67% of the 7315 respondents indicated that they were *somewhat to extremely bothered* by excess fat under their chin or neck [3]. While neurotoxins and dermal fillers are commonly used to treat wrinkles, folds, and volume loss, until recently there was no minimally invasive non-surgical pharmacologic option for submental contouring. Liposuction, often performed in conjunction with a face and/or neck lift, and direct fat excision are common procedures for submental contouring. Although these procedures often yield excellent results, they are invasive, associated with potential complications or long recovery times, and may not be appropriate for all patients [4]. In 2015, an alternative and first-in-class injectable pharmacologic treatment (deoxycholic acid injection; studied as ATX-101 by Kythera Biopharmaceuticals, Inc.) was approved by the US Food and Drug Administration (KYBELLA®, Allergan) and Health Canada (BELKYRA™, Allergan) for *improvement in the appearance of moderate to severe convexity or fullness associated with SMF in adults* [5].

Injectable Fillers: Facial Shaping and Contouring, Second Edition.

Edited by Derek H. Jones and Arthur Swift.

© 2019 John Wiley & Sons Ltd. Published 2019 by John Wiley & Sons Ltd.

Companion website: www.wiley.com/go/jones/injectable_fillers

10.1 Overview of ATX-101 for Submental Contouring

ATX-101 has been extensively investigated in a global clinical development program that included 18 trials (four phase 3 trials) and over 2600 subjects, of whom over 1600 were treated with ATX-101 [6]. The results from these trials are summarized below.

10.1.1 Mechanism of Action of ATX-101

The adipocytolytic effect observed with compounded phosphatidylcholine/sodium deoxycholate was initially attributed to phosphatidylcholine, while deoxycholate was thought to serve as a solubilizing excipient. However, Rotunda and colleagues demonstrated in 2004 that sodium deoxycholate caused adipocytolysis while phosphatidylcholine inhibited the effect of deoxycholate [7]. Subsequent experiments showed that deoxycholate is highly protein bound, protein binding inhibits the activity of deoxycholate, and protein-rich tissues are less sensitive to the cytolyic effect of deoxycholate [8]. Thus, adipose tissue is more sensitive to the effects of deoxycholate compared with skin or muscle [8].

The mechanism of action of ATX-101 was explored in a phase 1 study in which ATX-101 (1–$8\,mg\,cm^{-2}$) was injected into abdominal fat followed by abdominoplasty at various time points and histologic evaluation of the excised tissue samples [6, 9]. Focal adipocyte lysis was noted within a day of ATX-101 injection. An expected local tissue response to adipocytolysis was observed, which consisted of neutrophils between days 1 and 3, followed by macrophage infiltration that cleared liberated lipids and cellular debris. By day 28, local inflammation was largely resolved and thickening of fibrous septa was observed, suggesting an increase in total collagen (neocollagenesis). Figure 10.1 illustrates the mechanism of action of ATX-101 for reduction of SMF [10].

10.1.2 Pharmacology, Pharmacokinetics, and Pharmacodynamics of ATX-101

The pharmacokinetics and pharmacodynamics of ATX-101 were characterized in two phase 1 trials in which ATX-101 ($2\,mg\,cm^{-2}$; total dose: $100\,mg$) was injected into either SMF or abdominal fat [11, 12]. ATX-101 injections resulted in a rapid increase in the plasma concentration of deoxycholic acid with levels returning to baseline within 12–24 hours. Across both trials, substantial intra- and inter-subject variability in the plasma concentration of deoxycholic acid was noted both before and after ATX-101 injection [11, 12]. Even at maximum values post-ATX-101 injection, plasma concentrations remained within the physiologic range for endogenous deoxycholic acid observed within the population. Following ATX-101 administration

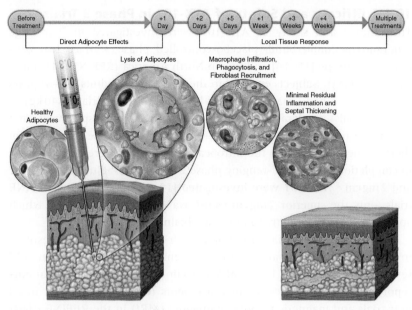

Figure 10.1 Mechanism of action of ATX-101.

and the resulting local adipocytolysis, plasma concentrations of total cholesterol, total triglycerides, and free fatty acids were comparable with those observed after a meal. There were no clinically meaningful changes in heart rate [11], other vital signs, or plasma levels of proinflammatory cytokines [12]. Furthermore, ATX-101 (100 mg and 200 mg) was shown to have no effect on QT/QTc intervals and was not associated with any cardiac safety signals [6].

10.1.3 Dose Optimization of ATX-101 for Submental Contouring

The optimal dose and treatment paradigm for submental contouring with ATX-101 was thoroughly investigated in three phase 2 trials in which multiple concentrations ($5–20$ mg ml^{-1}), injection volumes (0.2 or 0.4 ml), and physical spacing between injections (0.7-cm or 1.0-cm grid) were evaluated [6, 13, 14]. Efficacy was consistently greater with an area-adjusted dose of 2 mg cm^{-2} (achieved by administering 10 mg/mL ATX-101 via 0.2 ml injections on a 1-cm grid) compared with the 1 mg cm^{-2} dose. However, treatment with area-adjusted doses >2 mg cm^{-2}, either by increasing the concentration of ATX-101 or reducing the physical spacing between injections, resulted in more severe and longer duration adverse events (AEs) while not substantially improving efficacy [6].

10.1.4 Efficacy and Safety of ATX-101 in Phase 3 Trials

The efficacy and safety of ATX-101 were investigated in four large randomized, double-blind, placebo-controlled phase 3 trials, two conducted in Europe [15, 16] and two in North America (REFINE-1 [17] and REFINE-2 [18]). Subjects enrolled in these trials were adults (18–65 years of age) with a body mass index $\leq 30\,kg\,m^{-2}$ (European trials)/$\leq 40\,kg\,m^{-2}$ (REFINE trials), moderate or severe SMF (grade 2 or 3, respectively, on a validated 5-point scale [0–4]), and were dissatisfied with the appearance of their submental region. In the European trials, which were initiated prior to completion of the dose-ranging phase 2 trials, area-adjusted doses of 1 and $2\,mg\,cm^{-2}$ ATX-101 were investigated [15, 16], while in the REFINE trials, only the superior $2\,mg\,cm^{-2}$ dose was studied [17, 18], for which approval was subsequently sought and obtained [5].

In all four phase 3 trials, treatment with $2\,mg\,cm^{-2}$ ATX-101 resulted in clinically meaningful and statistically significant improvement in SMF severity assessed using both validated clinician-reported and patient-reported scales and objective measurements (calliper assessment in all four trials and magnetic resonance imaging (MRI) in the REFINE trials) [15–18]. In addition, patient satisfaction was high and the psychological impact of SMF was clinically meaningfully reduced following ATX-101 treatment [15–18]. In the four trials, all efficacy endpoints (assessed 12 weeks after last treatment) were met with statistical significance. Clinically meaningful improvement in SMF severity was reported in most ATX-101–treated subjects within two to four treatment sessions [17, 18]. In the European trials, consistently better efficacy was reported with the $2\,mg\,cm^{-2}$ dose of ATX-101 compared with the $1\,mg\,cm^{-2}$ dose [15, 16]. Representative before/after photographs coupled with MRI scans of an ATX-101–treated subject from the REFINE-1 trial are shown in Figure 10.2 [17].

Pain, swelling/oedema, bruising, numbness, erythema, and induration were commonly reported local AEs associated with ATX-101 treatment [15–18].These injection-site AEs, which were mostly mild/moderate, and transient, were expected based on the mechanism of action of ATX-101, the injection procedure, and the expected local tissue response. Incidences of marginal mandibular nerve paresis, skin ulceration, and dysphagia were low, mostly mild or moderate, and resolved without sequelae in all cases.

Skin laxity is a potential concern in the context of targeted fat reduction. In the phase 3 trials, >90% of ATX-101-treated subjects had unchanged or improved skin laxity from baseline despite significant reduction in SMF [15–18]. This may be due to the increase in total collagen (neocollagenesis) and tissue retraction observed with ATX-101 injections [6, 9], and suggests that additional procedures for skin tightening may not be necessary in patients treated with ATX-101.

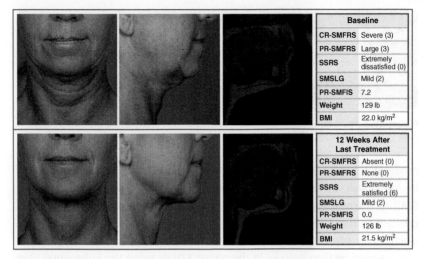

	Baseline
CR-SMFRS	Severe (3)
PR-SMFRS	Large (3)
SSRS	Extremely dissatisfied (0)
SMSLG	Mild (2)
PR-SMFIS	7.2
Weight	129 lb
BMI	22.0 kg/m²

	12 Weeks After Last Treatment
CR-SMFRS	Absent (0)
PR-SMFRS	None (0)
SSRS	Extremely satisfied (6)
SMSLG	Mild (2)
PR-SMFIS	0.0
Weight	126 lb
BMI	21.5 kg/m²

Figure 10.2 Standardized photographs and magnetic resonance images of a 50-year-old female patient who underwent five treatment sessions with ATX-101 and achieved a two-grade improvement in composite CR-SMFRS/PR-SMFRS response rates at 12 weeks after the last treatment. Percentage reduction in submental volume as assessed by MRI was 22.4%. BMI, body mass index; CR-SMFRS, Clinician-Reported Submental Fat Rating Scale; PR-SMFIS, Patient-Reported Submental Fat Impact Scale; PR-SMFRS, Patient-Reported Submental Fat Rating Scale; SMSLG, Submental Skin Laxity Grade; SSRS, Subject Self-Rating Scale.

10.1.5 Long-term Efficacy and Safety of ATX-101

SMF reduction with ATX-101 treatment is anticipated to be durable since ATX-101 destroys adipocytes. Long-term follow-up of treatment responders from phase 2/3 trials show that the majority maintain the treatment effect over time (with current data available for up to four years after treatment) [19]. AEs were uncommon during follow-up, and no new or unexpected safety concerns were identified [19].

10.2 Considerations for ATX-101 Treatment in Clinical Practice

10.2.1 Patient Selection and Evaluation

A key component of successful treatment with facial injectables is appropriate patient selection. During the initial consultation, a static as well as a dynamic assessment should be conducted, including a thorough physical examination and observation of the face and submental region from various angles. Using palpation, SMF (and not other conditions such as thyromegaly or cervical lymphadenopathy) should be identified as the

...

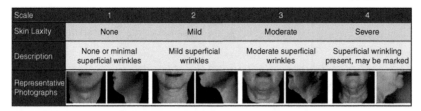

Scale	1	2	3	4
Skin Laxity	None	Mild	Moderate	Severe
Description	None or minimal superficial wrinkles	Mild superficial wrinkles	Moderate superficial wrinkles	Superficial wrinkling present, may be marked
Representative Photographs				

Figure 10.3 Photonumeric guide for assessment of skin laxity using the Submental Skin Laxity Grade Scale.

cause of submental fullness. As ATX-101 is meant to treat preplatysmal fat, the physician should confirm that the patient has enough preplatysmal SMF to warrant injection with ATX-101.Instructing patients to animate/grimace so that the platysma muscle is tensed/activated can also assist in isolating the preplatysmal fat. Features such as excessive skin laxity (which was assessed by the clinician in the phase 3 trials using the Submental Skin Laxity Gradescale (Figure 10.3) [17]) or presence of prominent platysmal bands that could lead to suboptimal results following SMF reduction, need to be taken into consideration prior to treatment. ATX-101 should not be administered to patients with infection in the treatment area. In patients with a history of dysphagia, ATX-101 injections may lead to swelling that may exacerbate the condition. Physicians should ensure that they have accurate information on previous aesthetic procedures, and the history of conditions such as injury to the marginal mandibular nerve, and baseline asymmetric smile/facial asymmetry.

ATX-101 is approved for use in adults 18–65 years of age [5]. A phase 3b trial investigating the safety and efficacy of ATX-101 treatment in subjects 65–75 years was recently completed (NCT02123134); however, results have not yet been published. In the meantime, ATX-101 should be used cautiously in older patients after taking into consideration their overall health and comorbidities. ATX-101 is approved for use in patients with moderate or severe SMF [5]. A phase 3b trial investigating the safety and efficacy of ATX-101 treatment in subjects with mild or extreme SMF was also recently completed (NCT02035267). Data from these trials will help further characterize the appropriate patient population for submental contouring with ATX-101.

10.2.2 Anatomy of the Submental Region

To avoid injuries to structures adjacent to the treatment area, knowledge of facial anatomy is crucial when injecting ATX-101. ATX-101 injections are administered in the submental region, which is bordered anteriorly by the submental crease and posteriorly by the hyoid bone. The lateral borders can be broadly defined by the caudal continuation of the labio-mandibular folds (Figure 10.4); however, SMF often extends beyond this

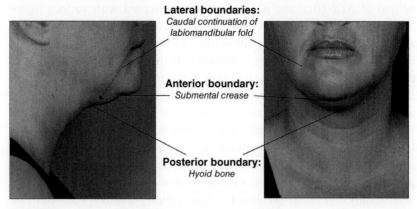

Lateral boundaries:
Caudal continuation of labiomandibular fold

Anterior boundary:
— *Submental crease* —

Posterior boundary:
Hyoid bone

Figure 10.4 Anatomic boundaries of the submental region.

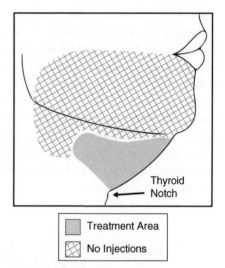

Thyroid
◄— Notch

Figure 10.5 Graphic representation of the treatment area, avoiding potential injury to the marginal mandibular nerve.

▢ Treatment Area

▨ No Injections

margin (especially in patients with larger necks or a wide distribution of SMF) and the lateral treatment areas can be defined on a case-by-case basis by clinical examination and palpation. ATX-101 injections should not be administered near the marginal mandibular branch of the facial nerve ('No injections'), which is the area above a line 1.0–1.5 cm inferior to the mandibular border from the gonium to the mentum (Figure 10.5) [5].

10.2.3 ATX-101 Injection Technique

Since appropriate administration of facial injectables is paramount to satisfactory outcomes, Kythera Biopharmaceuticals, Inc. facilitated an injection practicum and roundtable discussion with six experienced plastic surgeons and cosmetic dermatologists [20]. Using fresh-frozen cadavers and methylene blue dye (whose concentration and viscosity was matched to that of ATX-101), the participants experimented with various injection techniques. For optimal delivery of ATX-101, it was determined that ATX-101 injections should be administered perpendicular to the skin, midway into the preplatysmal fat, while keeping the preplatysmal fat pinched between two fingers (Figure 10.6) [20]. Tailoring the injections to the SMF thickness of an individual patient was determined to be more appropriate than defining arbitrary needle lengths for penetration into the skin. Injections that were too superficial (e.g. those administered while pinching the skin instead of subcutaneous fat) would lead to ATX-101 being deposited too close to the dermis, which could result in skin ulceration. Participants also evaluated the effect of pressure and injection volume on diffusion. A slow and steady pressure (vs. low or high pressures) resulted in an even distribution of ATX-101 in the preplatysmal fat. Injection volumes of 0.2 ml resulted in an area of diffusion of 15 mm, while volumes of 0.1 ml and 0.4 ml resulted in diffusion areas covering 10 and 30 mm, respectively. These findings are in line with the results from a porcine study in which the cytolytic effect of 0.2 ml injections of 10 mg ml^{-1} ATX-101 was most intense at the immediate point of injection, then diminished in a gradient fashion, with sparse cytolytic/apoptotic effects noted up to a maximum of 1.0–1.5 cm from the injection site [6]. These results, in conjunction with the results from the phase 2 dose optimization studies demonstrate that ATX-101 should be administered at an area-adjusted dose of 2 mg cm^{-2} as 0.2 ml injections of 10 mg ml^{-1} ATX-101 on a 1-cm grid to achieve even distribution of drug and to avoid dimpling or unevenness of results (Video 10.1) [20].

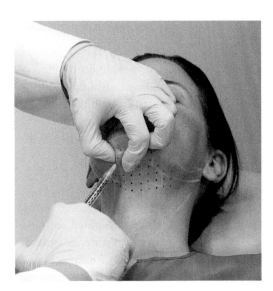

Figure 10.6 When administering ATX-101, physicians should pinch the fat between two fingers, pull it away from the underlying tissue, and inject perpendicular to the skin until the needle is midway into the underlying preplatysmal fat.

10.2.4 **Administration of ATX-101 Treatment**

Prior to starting ATX-101 treatment, the lower face and anterior neck are cleaned with a topical anaesthetic and the borders of the treatment area and the 'No Treatment Zone' are marked with a white marking pencil (Figure 10.7) [20]. Lidocaine-epinephrine injections can be administered (if needed) followed by application of the injection grid, and a cold pack is applied to the treatment area for approximately five minutes prior to injection. ATX-101 injections should be administered with a 30G (or smaller) 0.5-in. needle near, but not into grid markings (to prevent potential tattooing of the skin) (Figure 10.8) [20]. Unlike the procedure with many dermal fillers, ATX-101 is delivered as a depot into the subcutaneous fat, and the needle should not be withdrawn during injection as this could result in deposition of product into the dermis, with the potential for skin ulceration.

The volume of ATX-101 injected in a single treatment session is tailored to suit patient needs and is dependent on the amount and distribution of SMF and the patient's aesthetic goals. While a maximum of 10 ml can be injected [5], typical volumes injected in clinical practice are expected to be in the 3–5 ml range. The number of treatment sessions can also be individualized. Whereas patients can undergo a maximum of six treatment sessions (at least one month apart), most patients in clinical practice can expect to see SMF reduction within two to four treatment sessions. It is also expected that with subsequent treatment sessions, a lower volume

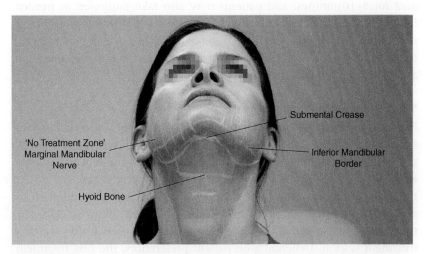

Figure 10.7 Pretreatment markings of the planned treatment area (corresponding to the submental fat compartment (bordered by the submental crease anteriorly, the hyoid bone posteriorly, and the caudal continuation of the labiomandibular folds laterally)) and the 'No Treatment Zone' (corresponding to the potential location of the marginal mandibular nerve).

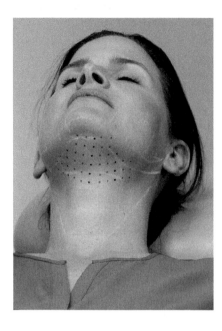

Figure 10.8 Illustration of 1.0-cm injection grid applied prior to treatment with ATX-101.

of ATX-101 would need to be administered due to the treatment effect of previous ATX-101 injections (reduction of target SMF). At the start of each treatment session, the physician should confirm the presence of sufficient SMF to warrant treatment.

Once treatment is completed, a cold pack can be applied to the treatment area for 5–10 minutes, and patients may also take ibuprofen as needed for up to three days. Patients should be assessed (both before and after treatment) for marginal mandibular nerve injury by checking the symmetry of their smile and for dysphagia, which could be a temporary sensation associated with post-treatment swelling.

10.2.5 Patient Management

Patient comfort and management play an important role in overall patient satisfaction, which, in turn, is an integral component of successful aesthetic treatments. During the initial consultation, patients should be thoroughly educated on the AEs associated with ATX-101 treatment as well as the time course for recovery from these events. Injection-site AEs such as pain, bruising, swelling, and numbness are expected following ATX-101 treatment, and typically decrease in incidence and severity after the first treatment session. Depending on patient preferences, the first treatment session should preferably be scheduled to allow sufficient time before resuming work or social activities (e.g. on a Monday or Friday afternoon).

An exploratory phase 3b study investigating interventions for management of common expected local injection-site AEs reported with ATX-101 treatment such as pain, swelling, and bruising showed that the these AEs are readily managed by physicians and tolerated by patients [21]. Pretreatment with cold/ice, topical lidocaine, and injectable lidocaine containing epinephrine decreased peak pain that occurred within the first five minutes following injection of ATX-101 by 17% compared with cold application alone. Further addition of loratadine and ibuprofen to this regimen resulted in total peak pain reduction by 40% compared with cold application alone. Bruising was mitigated to a modest extent by the vasoconstrictor effect of epinephrine and there was no indication of worsening of bruising with oral ibuprofen taken 30–60 minutes before injection [21].

In clinical practice, injectable lidocaine containing epinephrine is considered an important tool in patient management, and many physicians use a combination of injectable lidocaine, ibuprofen, and cold application for effective pain control. Lidocaine can be administered using multiple subcutaneous injections or through a single port using a microcannula. It is important to note that ATX-101 should not be administered using a cannula.

10.3 Summary

ATX-101 is a first-in-class injectable drug approved for non-surgical submental contouring. ATX-101 ($10 \, mg \, ml^{-1}$) is administered into the preplatysmal SMF as 0.2 ml injections spaced 1 cm apart. Although a maximum of 10 ml ATX-101 could be administered in a single treatment session and up to a maximum of six treatment sessions (spaced one month apart) were permitted in clinical trials, most patients in clinical practice are likely to see a gradual reduction in their SMF over a series of two to four treatment sessions, typically with 2–5 ml administered per treatment session. The common and expected local injection-site AEs reported with ATX-101 are typically mild/moderate, transient, do not cause patients to discontinue treatment, and are easily managed. Given this favourable risk : benefit profile, both physician and patient can have an ongoing dialogue regarding treatment and expectations. ATX-101 is a novel non-surgical tool available to physicians to sculpt/contour the submental region that results in high patient satisfaction.

10.3.1 Clinical Pearls

10.3.1.1 Pearl 1

At the initial consultation, it is important to counsel the patient regarding expectations, including the likely number of treatment sessions the patient will need for optimal results. Most patients will benefit from two to four sessions, but some patients could require more or less treatment sessions depending on their degree of SMF and treatment goals. It is helpful to show the patient before/after photographs of patients treated with ATX-101 and specify how many treatment sessions were required to achieve the results.

10.3.1.2 Pearl 2
As part of the initial consultation, it is necessary to discuss that some swelling will occur after each treatment session. Photographs of post-treatment swelling can help the patient visualize the swelling and demonstrate how the swelling is most significant in the first few days to 1 week, but gradually resolves. In rare instances, swelling may last several weeks. It is likely that patients will experience less swelling with each treatment session, but this is not always the case.

10.3.1.3 Pearl 3
Prior to treatment, patients should be aware of the potential complications of ATX-101. Aside from swelling, patients could experience bruising or numbness at the injection sites. Male patients should be aware that transient patchy alopecia may occur at an injection site. All patients should be warned of the risk for marginal mandibular nerve injury, which could result in a temporary asymmetric smile. Patients should be reassured that this complication is rare and all reported cases of nerve injury have resolved.

10.3.1.4 Pearl 4
Before each treatment, three-view 2-D or 3-D photographs should be taken of the patient. It is important that the patient is not smiling and that the chin is positioned at a 90°angle in the Frankfort plane to obtain an accurate and consistent view of SMF. These photographs will help the patient appreciate the improvement achieved with each treatment session.

10.3.1.5 Pearl 5
Prior to placement of the grid and/or injection with optional injectable anaesthesia, draw out the treatment area using a white marking pencil. The authors prefer to mark the patient prior to injection of anaesthesia as the swelling from the anaesthesia often distorts the anatomy. The treatment area is bordered by the submental crease, the hyoid bone, and the caudal continuation of the labiomandibular folds bilaterally in most patients, but should be tailored to the individual patient. Additionally, it can be helpful to mark an 'x' over the vicinity of the marginal mandibular nerve to make sure this area is not treated. Injections above 1 inch below the inferior border of the mandible, particularly in lateral regions, should be avoided to avoid potential marginal mandibular nerve injury.

10.3.1.6 Pearl 6
When anaesthetizing and treating the patient, it is preferred to have the patient in a reclined position at approximately 45° to provide a more natural angle to inject perpendicularly to the skin.

10.3.1.7 Pearl 7
It is important to manage discomfort and this can be accomplished using multiple modalities. Many physicans use lidocaine with epinephrine prior to the procedure to minimize pain and possibly reduce bruising; however, one of the authors does not typically use lidocaine. If lidocaine is used, it can be administered with multiple injections. One author uses a cannula and has found this technique to be effective. In the authors' experience, ice or cool air, acetaminophen, and non-steroidal anti-inflammatory drugs (NSAIDs) can reduce pain. Acetaminophen and NSAIDs can be administered 30 minutes prior to the procedure and continued as needed post-procedure.

10.3.1.8 Pearl 8
After marking the treatment area and anaesthetizing the patient, an injection grid is placed over the area. By counting the dots from the grid that fall inside the treatment area, one can estimate the volume of ATX-101 necessary for the treatment (0.2 ml of ATX-101 will be injected near each dot). The number of injection sites is divided by 5 to determine the volume of ATX-101 in 1.0-ml syringes needed for the treatment.

10.3.1.9 Pearl 9
ATX-101 can be drawn up into multiple 1.0-ml syringes and injected with 30–32G, 0.5-inch needles. In general, 0.2 ml of ATX-101 is injected near each dot within the treatment area. Some physicians may choose to inject 0.1 ml of ATX-101 in the most peripheral injection sites to taper the amount of ATX-101 injected to the area. The depth of the injections commonly range from 0.25 to 0.5 inch depending on the depth of SMF. Some practitioners may find it advantageous to have an assistant to hand them the needles and to help call out coloured dots and the number of syringes during treatment.

10.3.1.10 Pearl 10
After treatment is completed, ice should be provided immediately to relieve any potential discomfort. The peak discomfort associated with treatment typically occurs just as the injection procedure is completed. One author has found that some patients appreciate pressure support post-treatment, which can be provided by affixing a strip of Hypafix® tape under the chin, though a small study of chin straps found no reduction of swelling or pain. A follow-up appointment after six weeks or longer for photographs, re-evaluation, and possible re-treatment can be made.

10.4 Acknowledgement

Medical writing assistance was provided by Meenakshi Subramanian, PhD, CMPP, and Karen Stauffer, PhD, CMPP, of Evidence Scientific Solutions, Philadelphia, Pennsylvania, USA, and supported by Kythera Biopharmaceuticals, Inc., Westlake Village, California, USA.

References

1. American Society of Plastic Surgeons. Chin Surgery Skyrockets Among Women and Men in All Age Groups (press release). 2012 [accessed 7 June 2016]; Available from: https://www.plasticsurgery.org/news/press-releases/chin-surgery-skyrockets-among-women-and-men-in-all-age-groups.
2. Ellenbogen, R. and Karlin, J.V. (1980). Visual criteria for success in restoring the youthful neck. *Plast. Reconstr. Surg.* 66 (6): 826–837.
3. American Society for Dermatologic Surgery. Consumer Survey on Cosmetic Dermatologic Procedures. 2015 [cited 2016 June 7]; Available from: https://www.asds.net/_Media.aspx?id=8963.
4. Koehler, J. (2009). Complications of neck liposuction and submentoplasty. *Oral Maxillofac. Surg. Clin, North Am.* 21 (1): 43–52.
5. Kythera Biopharmaceuticals, Inc. KYBELLA (deoxycholic acid) injection [prescribing information]. April 30, 2015 [cited 2016 June 7]; Available from: http://consumers.mykybella.com/~/media/Unique%20Sites/Kybella/Documents/KYBELLA-Combined-FINAL-Labeling.ashx.
6. Kythera Biopharmaceuticals, Inc. Dermatologic and Ophthalmic Drugs Advisory Committee Briefing Document: ATX-101 (deoxycholic acid) injection. February 3, 2015 [accessed 18 September 2018]; Available from: https://www.accessdata.fda.gov/drugsatfda_docs/nda/2015/206333Orig1s000MedR.pdf.
7. Rotunda, A.M., Suzuki, H., Moy, R.L., and Kolodney, M.S. (2004). Detergent effects of sodium deoxycholate are a major feature of an injectable phosphatidylcholine formulation used for localized fat dissolution. *Dermatol. Surg.* 30 (7): 1001–1008.
8. Thuangtong, R., Bentow, J.J., Knopp, K. et al. (2010). Tissue-selective effects of injected deoxycholate. *Dermatol. Surg.* 36 (6): 899–908.
9. Walker P., Lee D., and Toth B.A. A histological analysis of the effects of single doses of ATX-101 on subcutaneous fat: results from a phase 1 open-label safety study of ATX-101 (abstract). Annual Meeting of the American Society for Dermatologic Surgery (3–6 October 2013), Chicago, IL.
10. Dayan, S.H., Humphrey, S., Jones, D.H. et al. (2016). Overview of ATX-101 (deoxycholic acid injection): a nonsurgical approach for reduction of submental fat. *Dermatol. Surg.* 42 (Suppl. 1): S263–S270.
11. Walker, P., Fellmann, J., and Lizzul, P.F. (2015). A phase I safety and pharmacokinetic study of ATX-101: injectable, synthetic deoxycholic acid for submental contouring. *J. Drugs Dermatol.* 14 (3): 279–284.
12. Walker, P. and Lee, D. (2015). A phase I pharmacokinetic study of ATX-101: serum lipids and adipokines following synthetic deoxycholic acid injections. *J. Cosmet. Dermatol.* 14 (1): 33–39.

13. Goodman, G., Smith, K., Walker, P., and Lee, D. (2012). Reduction of submental fat with ATX-101: a pooled analysis of two international multicenter, double-blind, randomized, placebo-controlled studies. *J. Am. Acad Dermatol* 66 (4 Suppl. 1): AB23.

14. Dover, J., Schlessinger, J., Young, L., and Walker, P. (2012). Reduction of submental fat with ATX-101: results from a phase IIB study using investigator, subject, and magnetic resonance imaging assessments. *J. Am. Acad Dermatol.* 2 (4 Suppl. 1): AB29.

15. Ascher, B., Hoffmann, K., Walker, P. et al. (2014). Efficacy, patient-reported outcomes and safety profile of ATX-101 (deoxycholic acid), an injectable srug for the reduction of unwanted submental fat: results from a phase III, randomized, placebo-controlled study. *J. Eur. Acad. Dermatol. Venereol.* 28 (12): 1707–1715.

16. Rzany, B., Griffiths, T., Walker, P. et al. (2014). Reduction of unwanted submental fat with ATX-101 (deoxycholic acid), an adipocytolytic injectable treatment: results from a phase III, randomized, placebo-controlled study. *Br. J. Dermatol* 170 (2): 445–453.

17. Jones, D.H., Carruthers, J., Joseph, J.H. et al. (2016). REFINE-1, a multicenter, randomized, double-blind, placebo-controlled, phase 3 trial with ATX-101, an injectable drug for submental fat reduction. *Dermatol. Surg.* 42 (1): 38–49.

18. Humphrey, S., Sykes, J., Kantor, J. et al. (2016). ATX-101 for reduction of submental fat: a phase III randomized controlled trial. *J. Am. Acad. Dermatol.* 75 (4): 788–797.

19. Bhatia A.C., Dayan S.H., Hoffmann K., Rubin M.G., Goodman G., Gross T.M., et al., eds. Reductions in submental fat achieved with deoxycholic acid injection (ATX-101) are maintained over time: results from long-term, follow-up studies (abstract). Annual Meeting of the American Society for Dermatologic Surgery (15–18 October 2015), Chicago, IL.

20. Jones, D.H., Kenkel, J.M., Fagien, S. et al. (2016). Proper technique for administration of ATX-101 (deoxycholic acid injection): insights from an injection practicum and roundtable discussion. *Dermatol. Surg* 42 (Suppl. 11): S275–S281.

21. Dover, J.S., Kenkel, J.M., Carruthers, A. et al. (2016). Management of patient experience with ATX-101 (deoxycholic acid injection) for reduction of submental fat. *Dermatol. Surg.* 42 (Suppl. 1): S288–S299.

CHAPTER 11

Avoidance and Management of Complications

Katie Beleznay[1] and Derek H. Jones[2]

[1] Carruthers & Humphrey Cosmetic Dermatology and University of British Columbia, Vancouver, British Columbia, Canada
[2] Skin Care and Laser Physicians of Beverly Hills, Los Angeles, CA, USA

11.1 Introduction

Injection of soft tissue fillers is one of the most common cosmetic procedures performed worldwide. Their popularity is partly due to their favourable side-effect profile. However, complications can occur and it is important for injecting physicians to have a firm knowledge of these complications to both prevent and manage adverse events (Table 11.1).

11.2 Early Injection Site Reactions

Injection site reactions are common and include erythema, swelling, pain, and bruising. These reactions typically resolve within one to two weeks. Strategies to minimize these risks include reducing the number of skin punctures and applying ice [1]. Bruising can be limited by avoiding blood-thinning medications or supplements for at least 7–10 days prior to injection. Using a small gauge needle, blunt cannula, and injecting small volumes slowly can further reduce bruising. However, despite even the best techniques, bruising may occur. Bruising can be treated with intense pulsed light, potassium titanyl phosphate (KTP), or pulsed dye lasers (Figure 11.1), which target the extravasated haemoglobin as a chromophore [2]. Superficial bruising from fillers will often lighten significantly within a day following laser or light-based treatment.

Injectable Fillers: Facial Shaping and Contouring, Second Edition.
Edited by Derek H. Jones and Arthur Swift.
© 2019 John Wiley & Sons Ltd. Published 2019 by John Wiley & Sons Ltd.
Companion website: www.wiley.com/go/jones/injectable_fillers

Table 11.1 Filler complications.

Type	Description
Early injection site reactions	Erythema, swelling, pain, and bruising
Technique and placement related	Nodules, beading, Tyndall effect
Delayed Nodules	Infectious, biofilms, granulomas, inflammatory/ immune-mediated
Vascular	Skin necrosis, blindness

(a) (b)

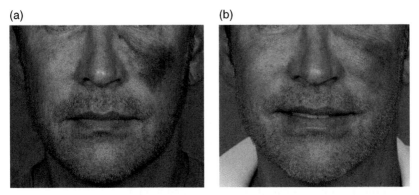

Figure 11.1 (a) Dense traumatic purpura of >10 days duration; (b) two days after treatment of purpura with a pulsed-dye laser.

11.3 Technique and Placement Related Complications

Inappropriate placement of fillers may result in palpable nodules and papules. Further, injecting too superficially with a hyaluronic acid (HA) filler may lead to beading or a blue-grey discoloration secondary to the Tyndall effect. This effect, if resulting from an HA filler, can be treated with hyaluronidase (Figure 11.2). Synthetic and permanent fillers can lead to persistent papules or nodules, particularly if they are placed too superficially in certain locations (Figures 11.3 and 11.4).

One advantage of HA fillers is that they are reversible and hyaluronidase can be used to treat complications. Juvederm® Ultra® is highly hydrophilic and should not be used in the tear trough or lid/cheek junction as delayed swelling may occur, even months or years post-treatment. The markings in Figure 11.5a outline the sausage-like swelling months after Juvederm Ultra injection. The markings post Vitrase® (Bausch and Lomb, Inc., Tampa, FL) (Figure 11.5b) indicate areas where a HA filler with a lower tendency for delayed swelling (Restlyane®, Belotero®, Volbella®) may be injected. Figure 11.6 shows a lip nodule from HA filler before (a) and after (b) treatment with Vitrase. Vitrase and Hylenex® (Halozyme Therapeutics,

(a)   (b)

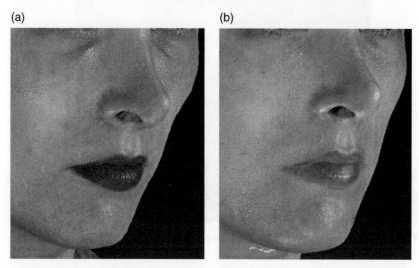

Figure 11.2 (a) Tyndall effect post HA filler in the tear trough; (b) Tyndall effect resolved post hyaluronidase.

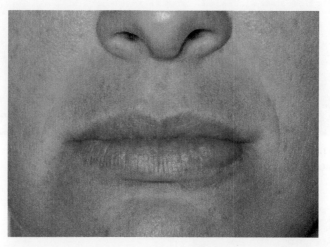

Figure 11.3 Calcium hydroxylapatite (CaHA) lip nodule persistent two years after injection. CaHA should not be injected too superficially or into the lips.

Inc., San Diego, CA) are two FDA-approved formulations of hyaluronidase that may be used off-label to remove HA filler. Hylenex is a genetically engineered human recombinant hyaluronidase, whereas Vitrase is ovine testicular derived hyaluronidase [3]. Hyaluronidase can be used to dissolve filler to resolve papules, nodules, Tyndall effect, or vascular compromise.

An in vitro, dose–response study suggests that Juvederm is more resistant to hyaluronidase compared to Restylane® [4]. In the author's experience, 10 units of hyaluronidase (Vitrase) per $0.1 \, cm^3$ of Juvederm or 5 units

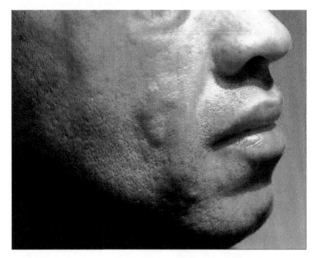

Figure 11.4 Silicone nodule secondary to superficial injection of liquid silicone.

(a)   (b)

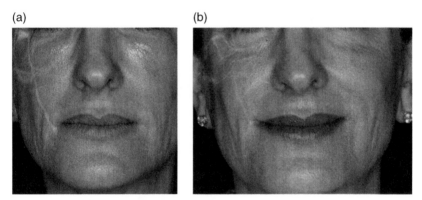

Figure 11.5 (a) Overfill of tear trough with Juvederm Ultra; (b) post-treatment with Vitrase for overfilled tear trough.

(a)

(b)

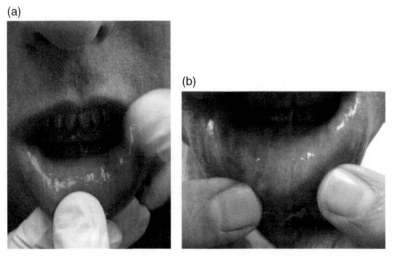

Figure 11.6 (a) Lip nodule from HA filler; (b) lip nodule resolved after treatment with Vitrase.

per 0.1 cm³ of Restylane may be the most appropriate dose to dissolve the HA. The need for more hyaluronidase for Juvederm is likely because the product is more highly cross linked [4]. In the case of impending necrosis, a minimum of 500 units of hyaluronidase should be used and the area should be retreated every 60–90 minutes until the ischemia resolves (skin colour and capillary refill return to normal) [5]. An abstract presented at the American Society for Dermatologic Surgery Annual Meeting in 2016 showed that in an in vivo rodent model there were no differences in hyaluronidase degradation of two HA fillers, Juvederm Ultra (24 mg/ml HA content with 0.3% lidocaine) or Voluma (20 mg/ml HA content with 0.3% lidocaine) when controlling for filler volume, depth, and location. The degree of degradation was dose dependent, as the lower doses of hyaluronidase maintained a higher level of filler projection. At the manufacturer-supplied concentrations, the source of hyaluronidase either Hylenex (recombinant human source) or Vitrase (ovine source) was interchangeable. Degradation was similar when hyaluronidase was administered (10 U/0.1 ml of filler) at four days or four weeks post-filler injection, indicating that tissue integration did not impede the ability of hyaluronidase to degrade HA filler [6].

The published incidence of allergic reaction to hyaluronidase is low at 1 per 1000 [5]. There is a theoretical cross-reactivity in patients who are allergic to honeybees and wasps, and patients who have had severe reactions or anaphylaxis to bee stings should be skin tested prior to non-emergent treatment with hyaluronidase [3]. For vascular compromise a skin test is not required, given the urgency of the situation, providing the patient does not have a known history of anaphylaxis. Treating physicians should be prepared for the very rare case of allergy or anaphylaxis [5].

11.4 Delayed Nodules

Delayed nodules secondary to filler have heterogeneous aetiologies and are difficult to definitively diagnose without histopathology or culture results. Delayed nodules may result from infections, biofilms, foreign body granulomas, or inflammatory/immune-mediated causes. Infection following filler treatment is uncommon, but can occur with any procedure that breaks the surface of the skin. Potential infectious aetiologies may be bacterial, fungal, or viral. To minimize the risk of infection, the skin should be cleansed prior to injection with an antimicrobial agent such as isopropyl alcohol or chlorhexidine. Chlorhexidine may be toxic to the cornea, and is best applied to the skin as a swab on gauze which may prevent splash injury to the eye. Techni-Care® is an alternative antiseptic which is safe to use around the eyes. The clinical presentation of infections may

(a)   (b)

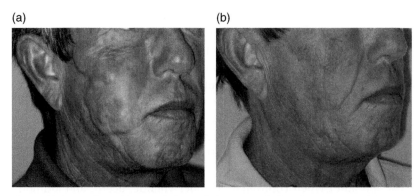

Figure 11.7 Bio-alcamid bacterial abscess before (a) and after (b) incision and drainage. Source: Reproduced with permission from [7].

include tender erythematous fluctuant nodules or abscesses. Figure 11.7 demonstrates a Bioalcamid bacterial abscess pre- and post-incision and drainage [8]. Systemic symptoms such as fever may occur, but are rare. A lesion suspected of having an infection should be cultured and/or biopsied. Treatment measures to consider include incision and drainage and/or broad-spectrum antibiotics such as clarithromycin until the culture results are back [9]. Trauma from the filler injection can also lead to reactivation of herpes virus infection. If the patient is receiving treatment in the perioral area and has a history of cold sores, prophylactic antiviral treatment should be considered [2].

Biofilms have implicated as one cause of delayed nodules after filler. Bacteria are thought to coat the filler when it is injected, forming a biofilm. Biofilms secrete a protective matrix that allows them to adhere to surfaces resulting in a low-grade chronic infection that is resistant to the immune system and antibiotics. Cultures are often negative as standard culturing techniques are not sensitive enough to detect the microorganisms [2]. To reduce the risk of acquiring biofilms, it is important to avoid any contamination during the implantation. Sterile technique should be used when reconstituting or diluting filler. Make-up and other potential contaminants on the skin should be removed, and an antimicrobial cleanser should be used prior to injection [10]. Given the challenge of culturing bacteria from biofilms and making a definitive diagnosis, many physicians recommend treating delayed nodules empirically with oral antibiotics such as clarithromycin for two to six weeks [2]. Foreign body granulomas are another potential cause of delayed nodules. Nodules may result from poly-L-lactic acid (PLLA) injection. Figure 11.8a reveals a granulomatous reaction caused by an injection of PLLA that was too superficial, while Figure 11.8b reveals a biopsy of the same, with a granulomatous infiltrate surrounding PLLA particles on histology. To avoid this reaction, PLLA should not

(a)   (b)

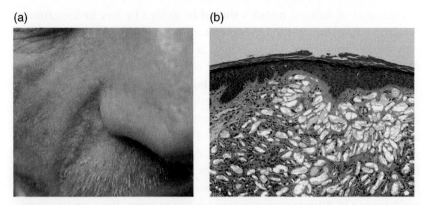

Figure 11.8 (a) Nodules resulting from poly-ʟ-lactic acid (PLLA) injection; (b) dermal granulomatous infiltrate surrounding PLLA particles. Haematoxylin–eosin stain, original magnification ×40. Source: Reproduced with permission from [11].

be injected intradermally [11]. Synthetic fillers can act as foreign bodies, stimulating a host response and granulomatous inflammation. This presentation, though rare, has been reported and confirmed with histology [2]. Granulomatous reactions may be seen more commonly with permanent fillers, and are best treated with combinations of $50\,mg/cm^3$ 5-fluorouracil admixed with 10% volume triamcinolone $40\,mg/cm^3$ [12].

Inflammatory or immune-mediated causes of delayed nodules have become increasingly recognized in the literature. HA fillers are not typically considered strongly immunostimulatory because HA is a natural component of the dermis and has no species specificity. However, both immediate and delayed hypersensitivity reactions have been described with HA fillers [13]. Time to onset of delayed nodules ranged from one month to three years after HA implantation [14]. It has been proposed that immune reactions could be due to residual proteins or impurities resulting from the manufacturing process; however, the manufacturing process has improved with time [9]. While HA injected on its own does not act as a foreign antigen, more recent data suggests that it has a larger role than an inert structural component. Data has shown that low-molecular weight HA (LMW-HA) is pro-inflammatory and can trigger the immune system [15]. This may be of particular importance in some of the delayed reactions seen with newer volumizing agents such as Juvederm® Voluma® XC (Vycross® technology, which also comprises Volift® and Vobella®). It is possible that as the filler breaks down, particularly over the three to five months post-injection, an increased exposure to LMW-HA fragments or catabolic by-products can stimulate an immune response. Having an inflammatory response to filler may be more common when the immune system is primed after a triggering event, such as a recent infection like influenza or a dental procedure [10].

Treatment of delayed nodules should be guided by any investigational results such as histopathology or culture. These inflammatory nodules may resolve spontaneously; however, removal of HA filler by hyaluronidase, or incision and drainage can be considered. Treatments that have been used for delayed nodules include but are not limited to: intralesional hyaluronidase; topical, oral, or intralesional corticosteroids; oral antibiotics; intralesional 5-fluorouracil; oral immunosuppressants; and lasers; or a combination of these treatments [9]. For delayed inflammatory events with HA (seen more frequently with Vycross technology), the authors' first line treatment approach includes watchful waiting, intralesional hyaluronidase (10 units of hyaluronidase per 0.1 cm³ of Juvederm), oral prednisone (20–40 mg every morning for five to seven days), and/or intralesional triamcinolone acetonide (5–10 mg per ml, with repeat injections at two to four weeks as needed). If a biofilm is suspected, clarithromycin 500 mg orally twice daily for two to six weeks can be used [10].

11.5 Vascular

The most serious potential complications from filler are vascular compromise with skin necrosis or blindness. To highlight the significance of this issue, the FDA issued a safety communication about the risk of intravascular injection with soft-tissue fillers [16]. Tissue necrosis may occur if filler is injected into blood vessels resulting in ischaemic or embolic phenomena (Figures 11.9 and 11.10). Blindness results from retrograde embolization of filler into the

(a)   (b)

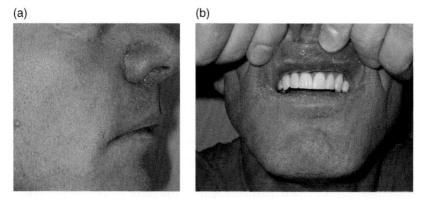

Figure 11.9 Vascular occlusion of the angular artery secondary to CaHA injection. Upon injection of the superior nasolabial fold with a needle, blanching was noted in the distribution of the angular artery. A tender pustular reaction developed within 24 hours (a) with mucosal sloughing apparent in the distribution of the superior labial artery secondary to the embolic phenomenon; (b) the adverse event resolved with no scarring or sequelae.

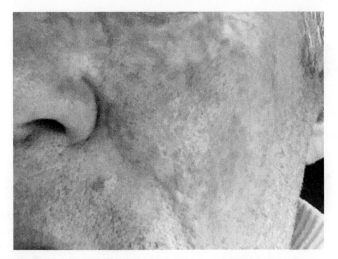

Figure 11.10 Upon injection of hyaluronic acid into the mid-cheek, immediate reticulated blanching was noted that resolved with massage. Within 24 hours, the patient presented with reticulated erythema as seen here; 100 units of Vitrase was injected at the suspected area of occlusion, with complete resolution of the skin changes within two days and no development of necrosis.

ocular vessels. Symptoms of vascular compromise include pain, blanching, duskiness, and reticulated violaceous erythema. This can progress to necrosis and scarring. Visual complications after filler may present with immediate unilateral vision loss, ocular pain, headache, nausea, or vomiting. Further, patients may have central nervous system complications including infarction and hemiplegia in association with blindness. In a recent review of the world literature there were 98 cases of blindness reported. Autologous fat was the most common filler type to cause this complication (nearly 48%) followed by HA (23.5%). The sites that were high risk for complications were the glabella (38.8%), nasal region (25.5%), nasolabial fold (13.3%), and forehead (12.2%), but virtually every anatomic location where filler is injected in the face is at risk for vascular compromise (Figure 11.11) [17].

11.5.1 Vascular Anatomy

Having a firm understanding of the vascular anatomy (Figure 11.12) prior to injection is critical to prevent these complications. Most of the blood supply to the face is through the external carotid artery, except for a region of the central face encompassing the eye, upper nose, and central forehead. The ophthalmic artery, a branch of the internal carotid, provides the blood supply to this area [18]. The ophthalmic artery branches into various arteries including the supraorbital, supratrochlear, and dorsal nasal artery. The facial artery branches off the external carotid artery. It passes over the jaw anterior to the masseter muscle and proceeds in

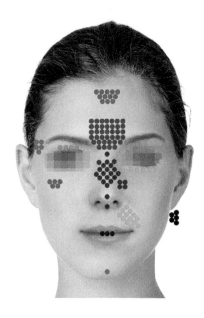

Figure 11.11 Location of injection for each case of blindness from filler. The five black dots represent cases in which the location was not specified and listed as 'face'. Source: Reproduced with permission from [17].

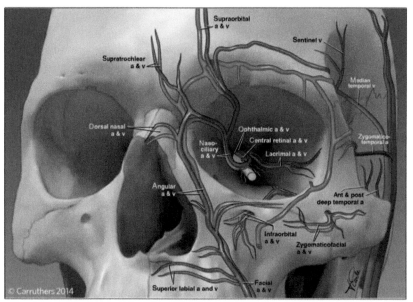

Figure 11.12 Vascular anatomy of the upper face: a, artery; v, vein. Source: Reproduced with permission from Jean D. Carruthers, MD, 2014 [17].

a superior and diagonal direction. The facial artery becomes known as the angular artery in the region of the nasolabial fold and has variable patterns as it continues superiorly. It anastomoses with other facial vessels including the dorsal nasal artery connecting the external and internal carotid system (Figure 11.13) [19].

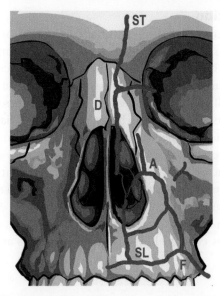

Figure 11.13 Vascular anatomy of the midface. The angular artery (a branch of the facial artery) anastomoses with the supratrochlear and dorsal nasal arteries (branches of the ophthalmic artery), joining the external carotid artery network with the internal carotid artery network. Occlusion or embolic events involving this network can lead to extensive tissue necrosis. A, angular artery; D, dorsal nasal artery; F, facial artery; SF, superior labial artery; ST, supratrochlear artery. Source: Reproduced with permission from Derek H. Jones.

It is important to understand the depth and location of vessels in high-risk sites. In the glabella and forehead the two major arteries are the supra-trochlear artery, which is found along the medial canthal vertical line, and supraorbital artery, which is more lateral in the region of the medial iris. Both of these arteries start their course deep and become more superficial approximately 15–20 mm above the supraorbital rim. They remain in the subcutaneous plane as they travel superiorly on the forehead. Therefore, injections at the levels of the supraorbital rim or within 2 cm of that location should be superficial. However, injections more superiorly on the forehead should be deep in a supraperiosteal plane [20]. In the nasal region there are many anastamotic vessels and therefore filler is most safely placed in the avascular deep supraperiosteal plane [21]. If the patient has had previous surgical procedures to the nose, filler injections should be avoided or carried out with extreme caution. The most likely blood vessel at risk for compromise in the medial cheek, nasolabial fold, and medial periorbital area is the angular artery. The angular artery can have variable patterns after it branches off the facial artery and can be located in the subcutaneous layer, so caution is advised when injecting in this region. With the rich vascular supply of the face and multiple anastomoses, it is very important to understand the location of vessels and appropriate depth of injection [17].

11.5.2 Prevention

Strategies to prevent vascular complications are critical, as we do not have well-documented successful treatment protocols. Most important is a firm understanding of the vascular anatomy and depth of injection, particularly in high risk sites such as the glabella, nasolabial fold, and nose. Choosing a reversible HA filler allows for treatment with hyaluronidase and the possibility of reversing vascular occlusion if used immediately when complications are noticed. Other strategies to implement include using low volumes of product, injecting slowly, and using a small gauge needle or cannula. Cannulae are blunt tipped and many believe that they reduce the risk of vascular injury, particularly in high-risk areas such as the cheek and nasolabial fold region medial to the mid-pupillary line. The author (DJ) demonstrates high-risk anatomy and the use of cannulas in the accompanying video to this chapter. Key prevention strategies are highlighted in Box 11.1.

Box 11.1 Key Strategies to Prevent Vascular Compromise

- Use a cannula as they are less likely to pierce a blood vessel. The authors in particular recommend using a cannula in the medial cheek, tear trough, and nasolabial fold.
- Before injecting, a detailed history should be obtained, including any previous cosmetic procedures or surgeries. Use extreme caution or avoid injecting a patient who has had a prior surgical procedure in the area.
- Know the location and depth of facial vessels and the common variations. Injectors should understand the appropriate depth and plane of injection at different sites.
- Choosing a reversible HA filler increases the likelihood of resolution without sequelae as hyaluronidase can be used to remove the product.
- Consider using a small diameter needle.* A smaller needle necessitates slower injection [23].
- Smaller syringes are preferred as larger syringes may make it more challenging to control the volume and increases the probability of injecting a larger bolus [24].
- Consider mixing the filler with epinephrine to promote vasoconstriction as cannulating a vasoconstricted artery is more difficult [23].
- Aspirate prior to injection. This recommendation is controversial as it may not be possible to get flashback into a syringe through fine needles with thick gels [25].
- Inject slowly and with minimal pressure.
- Inject in small increments to prevent a large column of filler travelling retrograde. No more than 0.1 ml of filler should be injected with each increment [23, 25].
- Move the needle tip during injection, so as not to deliver a large deposit in one location.

* For injection of autologous fat, many experts recommend using larger 16–18 gauge blunter cannulae as smaller sharp needles/cannulas are more likely to perforate blood vessels. The syringe size should be limited to 1 ml and less than 0.1 ml of autologous fat should be injected with each pass of the cannula [22].

11.5.3 Treatment

Treatment should be instituted immediately at the first sign of vascular compromise. It is important to recognize, however, that treatment recommendations are not based on a large body of evidence. The goal of treatment is rapid restoration of perfusion. Key management strategies for vascular compromise with skin sequelae (Box 11.2) [26] and ocular complications (Box 11.3) will be discussed.

If blanching occurs while injecting filler, immediately discontinue the injection. If the complication occurs with an HA filler, hyaluronidase is recommended. Different formulations are available, which makes it difficult to establish standardized dosing. Variable doses have been reported from 10 to 30 units per $2 \times 2\,cm^2$ area along the artery and its branches [26] up to 1500 units [27]. In addition, treatments that should be initiated include warm compresses and massage. Other potential therapies include topical nitroglycerine paste, aspirin, oral prednisone, hyperbaric oxygen, and low molecular weight heparin. A thorough individual assessment and

---

Box 11.2 Treatment of Vascular Compromise with Skin Sequelae

- Stop the injection immediately
- Inject hyaluronidase if an HA filler was used
- Apply warm compresses every 10 minutes for the first few hours
- Vigorous massage
- Consider applying topical 2% nitroglycerine paste
- Consider administering aspirin, 325 mg under tongue immediately and 81 mg daily thereafter
- Consider oral prednisone 20–40 mg daily for 3–5 days
- Consider hyperbaric oxygen
- Follow patient daily until improvement. Provide them with clear written treatment instructions

---

Box 11.3 Treatment of Vascular Compromise with Ocular Complications

- If symptoms of ocular pain or vision changes occur, stop the injection at once. Immediately contact an ophthalmologist or oculoplastics colleague and urgently transfer the patient directly there.
- Consider treating the injected area and surrounding location with hyaluronidase if a HA filler was used.
- Consider retrobulbar injection of 300–600 units (2–4 cm³) of hyaluronidase if a HA filler was used [27].
- Mechanisms to reduce intraocular pressure should be considered such as ocular massage, anterior chamber paracentesis, intravenous mannitol, and acetazolamide [23].

treatment plan with close follow-up should be initiated for each patient to ensure optimal outcomes [7].

Management of vascular compromise with subsequent blindness is more challenging as there are few reported successful treatments and no consistent evidence-based treatment strategies. In addition, there is a strict timeline, as after 90 minutes the damage secondary to the retinal ischaemia is more likely to be irreversible [28].

First and foremost, if the patient complains of ocular pain or vision changes, the injection should be stopped immediately. The patient should be immediately transferred to an ophthalmologist or oculoplastics colleague. One should consider injecting large volumes of hyaluronidase at the injection site and surrounding areas if an HA filler was used. It has been shown that hyaluronidase can diffuse through the blood vessel walls without needing to be directly injected into the vessel [25]. As such, if vision loss occurs after an HA filler, retrobulbar injection of hyaluronidase is a potential vision-saving treatment. Jean Carruthers first proposed an injection of 300–600 units of hyaluronidase into the retrobulbar space. The technique involves anaesthetizing an area over the lateral lower eyelid. A 25G needle is advanced at this location until it is at least 1 inch deep; 2–4 cm³ of hyaluronidase are then injected in the inferolateral orbit (please see Video 11.1 demonstrating retrobulbar injection) [28]. The successful restoration of visual loss with this technique has been reported [29]. Other treatments that have been tried include mechanisms to decrease intraocular pressure such as anterior chamber decompression, mannitol, and acetazolamide. Further strategies include hyperbaric oxygen, systemic and local intra-arterial fibrinolysis, and systemic corticosteroids; however, these treatments are not consistently successful [17].

11.6 Conclusion

As the use of soft tissue fillers continues to rise, it is important to be aware of possible complications. With appropriate knowledge, soft tissue augmentation is a highly effective and safe procedure. To minimize any adverse events, a thorough understanding of facial anatomy and proper injection technique is imperative. Injectors should be aware of both prevention and management strategies to minimize complications and improve patient outcomes.

References

1. Alam, M., Gladstone, H., Kramer, E.M. et al. (2008). ASDS guidelines of care: injectable fillers. *Dermatol. Surg.* 34 (Suppl. 1): S115–S148.
2. Funt, D. and Pavicic, T. (2013). Dermal fillers in aesthetics: an overview of adverse events and treatment approaches. *Clin. Cosmet. Investig. Dermatol.* 6: 295–316.

3. Keller, E.C., Kaminer, M.S., and Dover, J.S. (2014). Use of hyaluronidase in patients with bee allergy. *Dermatol. Surg.* 40: 1145–1147.

4. Jones, D., Tezel, A., and Borell, M. (2010). In-vitro resistance to degradation of HA by ovine testicular hyaluronidase. *Dermatol. Surg.* 36 (s1): 804–809.

5. DeLorenzi, C. (2017). New high dosed pulsed hyaluronidase protocol for hyaluronic acid filler vascular adverse events. *Aesthet Surg J.* 37: 814–825.

6. Shumate, G.T., Chopra, R., Jones, D. et al. (2018). In vivo degradation of crosslinked hyaluronic acid fillers by exogenous hyaluronidases. *Dermatol. Surg.* 44: 1075–1083.

7. Beleznay, K., Humphrey, S., Carruthers, J., and Carruthers, A. (2014). Vascular compromise from soft tissue augmentation: experience with 12 cases and recommendations for optimal outcomes. *J. Clin. Aesthet. Dermatol.* 7: 37–43.

8. Jones, D.H., Carruthers, A., Fitzgerald, R. et al. (2007). Late-appearing abscesses after injections of nonabsorbable hydrogel polymer for HIV-associated facial lipoatrophy. *Dermatol. Surg.* 33 (s2): S193–S198.

9. Glashofer, M.D. and Flynn, T.C. (2013). Complications of temporary fillers. In: *Soft Tissue Augmentation* (ed. J. Carruthers and A. Carruthers), 179–187. Toronto: Elsevier Saunders.

10. Beleznay, K., Carruthers, J.A., Carruthers, A. et al. (2015). Delayed-onset nodules secondary to a smooth cohesive 20 mg/mL hyaluronic acid filler: cause and management. *Dermatol. Surg.* 41: 929–939.

11. Wildemore, J. and Jones, D. (2006). Persistent granulomatous inflammatory response induced by poly-L-lactic acid for HIV lipoatrophy. *Dermatol. Surg.* 32: 1407–1409.

12. Jones, D. (2014). Treatment of delayed reactions to dermal fillers. *J. Dermatol. Surg.* 40 (11): 1180.

13. Alijotas-Reig, J., Fernandez-Figueras, M.T., and Puig, L. (2013). Inflammatory, immune-mediated adverse reactions related to soft tissue dermal fillers. *Semin. Arthritis. Rheum.* 43: 241–258.

14. Ledon, J.A., Savas, J.A., Yang, S. et al. (2013). Inflammatory nodules following soft tissue filler use: a review of causative agents, pathology and treatment options. *Am. J. Clin. Dermatol.* 14: 401–411.

15. Baeva, L.F., Lyle, D.B., Rios, M. et al. (2013). Different molecular weight hyaluronic acid effects on human macrophage interleukin 1B production. *J. Biomed. Mater. Res. A* 102A: 305–314.

16. Jagdeo, J. and Hruza, G. (2015). The Food and Drug Administration Safety Communication on Unintentional Injection of Soft-Tissue Filler into Facial Blood Vessels: Important Points and Perspectives. *Dermatol. Surg.* 41 (12): 1372–1374.

17. Beleznay, K., Carruthers, J., Humphrey, S., and Jones, D. (2015). Avoiding and treating blindness from fillers: a review of the world literature. *Dermatol. Surg.* 41: 1097–1117.

18. Larrabee, W.F., Makielski, K.H., and Henderson, J.L. (2004). *Surgical Anatomy of the Face*, 2e, 97–101. Philadelphia: Lippincott Williams & Wilkins.

19. Flowers, F.P. and Breza, T.S. (2012). Surgical anatomy of the head and neck. In: *Dermatology*, 3e (ed. J.L. Bolognia, J.L. Jorizzo and J.V. Schaffer), 2235–2236. China: Elsevier.

20. Kleintjes, W.G. (2007). Forehead anatomy: arterial variations and venous link of the midline forehead flap. *J. Plast. Reconstr. Aesthet. Surg.* 60: 593–606.

21. Saban, Y., Andretto Amodeo, C., Bouaziz, D. et al. (2012). Nasal arterial vasculature: medical and surgical applications. *Arch. Facial Plast. Surg.* 14: 429–436.

22. Yoshimura, K. and Coleman, S.R. (2015). Complications of fat grafting how they occur and how to find, avoid, and treat them. *Clin. Plast. Surg.* 42: 383–388.

23. Lazzeri, D., Agostini, T., Figus, M. et al. (2012). Blindness following cosmetic injections of the face. *Plast. Reconstr. Surg.* 129: 994–1012.

24. Coleman, S.R. (2002). Avoidance of arterial occlusion from injection of soft tissue fillers. *Aesthet. Surg. J.* 22: 555–557.

25. DeLorenzi, C. (2014). Complications of injectable fillers, part 2: vascular complications. *Aesthet. Surg. J.* 34: 584–600.

26. Dayan, S., Arkins, J.P., and Mathison, C.C. (2011). Management of impending necrosis associated with soft tissue filler injections. *J. Drugs Dermatol.* 10: 1007–1012.

27. DeLorenzi, C. (2013). Complications of injectable fillers, part I. *Aesthet. Surg. J.* 3: 561–575.

28. Carruthers, J.D., Fagien, S., Rohrich, R. et al. (2014). Blindness caused by cosmetic filler injection: a review of cause and therapy. *Plast. Reconst. Surg.* 134: 1197–1201.

29. Chestnut, C. (2018). Restoration of visual loss with retrobulbar hyaluronidase injection after hyaluronic acid filler. *Dermatol. Surg.* 44 (3): 435–437.

Index

Note: Page numbers in *italic* refer to figures. Page numbers in **bold** refer to tables.

Injectable Fillers: Facial Shaping and Contouring, Second Edition.
Edited by Derek H. Jones and Arthur Swift.
© 2019 John Wiley & Sons Ltd. Published 2019 by John Wiley & Sons Ltd.
Companion website: www.wiley.com/go/jones/injectable_fillers